NURSING HEALTH ASSESSMENT

Student Applications

Patricia M. Dillon, DNSc, RN
Adjunct Faculty
Temple University
College of Allied Health Professions
Department of Nursing
Philadelphia, Pennsylvania

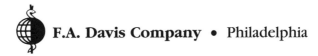
F.A. Davis Company • Philadelphia

F. A. Davis Company
1915 Arch Street
Philadelphia, PA 19103
www.fadavis.com

Printed in the United States of America

Last digit indicates print number: 10 9 8 7 6 5 4 3 2

Acquisitions Editor: Lisa B. Deitch
Cover Designer: Louis J. Forgione

As new scientific information becomes available through basic and clinical research, recommended treatments and drug therapies undergo changes. The author(s) and publisher have done everything possible to make this book accurate, up to date, and in accord with accepted standards at the time of publication. The author(s), editors, and publisher are not responsible for errors or omissions or for consequences from application of the book, and make no warranty, expressed or implied, in regard to the contents of the book. Any practice described in this book should be applied by the reader in accordance with professional standards of care used in regard to the unique circumstances that may apply in each situation. The reader is advised always to check product information (package inserts) for changes and new information regarding dose and contraindications before administering any drug. Caution is especially urged when using new or infrequently ordered drugs.

ISBN 0-8036-0890-X

Preface

Health assessment presents special challenges to learners, with its mass of detail that requires memorization, its organization that addresses each individual system but requires you to understand the whole, and its focus on the person as well as the body. We created this collection of activities, following the organization of the book *Nursing Health Assessment: A Critical Thinking, Case Studies Approach,* to enhance your learning of health assessment by:

- Providing anatomy and physiology review
- Defining a context within which you can apply assessment
- Reinforcing normal findings and selected abnormal findings
- Letting you have fun!

For each systems chapter, you will find the following:

- Normal anatomical structures that allow you to review anatomy
- A matching exercise that lets you review structure and function
- A short case study that provides a context in which you can apply assessment

  Notice that the case studies within the text allow you to focus on normal, whereas we designed the case studies in the workbook to allow you to differentiate normal from abnormal.

- Short-answer situational questions that facilitate your thinking and clinical decisions
- An exercise in which we ask you to identify the relationship of the system you're currently studying and all other systems (remember to look at a specific system as a part of the whole being)
- An abnormal case study that includes a health history, physical assessment, and questions to test your critical thinking skills
- Puzzles (word searches, jumbles) to reinforce assessment content.

  We hope you'll find these puzzles as fun to do as they were to create.

- A lab sheet, which covers history and physical findings and corresponds to the system chapter in the text

The history portion of the lab sheet addresses pertinent symptoms of the specific system, which you apply as they relate to that system. The physical assessment section of the lab sheet begins with a general survey and head-to-toe scan to identify the relationship of the particular system to other systems, then presents assessment of the system, techniques, client position, helpful hints in **bold**, alerts in ***bold italic***, the assessment, and normal findings with developmental and cultural variations in three columns. In the fourth column, which is blank, you can document your findings as you practice on other students in lab because just as you must develop your assessment skills, you must develop your documentation skills. Include negative findings in your documentation; this will help you to remember specifics of the assessment. At the end of the lab sheet, space is provided in which you can identify pertinent history and physical findings and formulate actual or potential nursing diagnoses. (Keep in mind that you can use lab sheets as a study aid, too!)

- A self-evaluation exercise in which we ask you to identify learning achieved and further learning needed

  Assessment is a skill; the more you practice, the better your skills become, and it is up to you to develop the skills and identify areas where you need more practice. Because you will be responsible and accountable for your practice and the patients you care for, so too you need to be accountable and responsible for your learning, tracking your progress and identifying further learning needs.

In Chapter 20, "Putting It All Together," complete health history and physical assessment forms are provided in which you can document your findings. We've also provided a guide "at a glance" for the health history and physical examination, which helps you perform a comprehensive systematic assessment by reminding you of questions to ask and the sequence of the examination.

Use these exercises to learn and reinforce your assessment skills. Remember, assessment is the first step of the nursing process, so make it count! Practice, practice, practice!

Contributors

Noreen Chikotas, MSN, CRNP
Assistant Professor
Department of Nursing
Bloomsburg University
Bloomsburg, Pennsylvania
Case study for Chapter 18. Assessing the Motor-
Musculoskeletal System

Denise Demers, RN, MS
Assistant Professor of Nursing
St. Joseph's College
Standish, Maine
Case study for Chapter 15. Assessing the
Abdomen

Pamela Jean Frable, ND, RN
Assistant Professor
Harris School of Nursing
Texas Christian University
Fort Worth, Texas
Case study for Chapter 4. Teaching the Client

Mary Jo Goolsby, MSN, EdD, ANP-C, FAANP
Director of Research and Education
American Academy of Nurse Practitioners
Austin, Texas
Patient Care Research Specialist
University Health Care System
Augusta, Georgia
Case study for Chapter 8. Assessing the
Integumentary System
Case study for Chapter 9. Assessing the Head,
Face, and Neck

Diane Greslick, RNc, MSN
Assistant Professor of Nursing
St. Joseph's College
Standish, Maine
Case study for Chapter 15. Assessing the
Abdomen

Annette Gunderman, RN, DEd
Associate Professor
Department of Nursing
Bloomsburg University

Bloomsburg, Pennsylvania
Case study for Chapter 18. Assessing the Motor-
Musculoskeletal System

Judith Ann Kilpatrick, RN, MSN, DNSc
Assistant Professor of Nursing
Widener University
Chester, Pennsylvania
Case study for Chapter 7. Spiritual Assessment

Carol Meadows, RNP, MNSc, APN
Instructor
University of Arkansas
Eleanor Mann School of Nursing
Fayetteville, Arkansas
Case study for Chapter 17. Assessing the Male
Genitourinary System
Case study for Chapter 24. Assessing the School-
Age Child and Adolescent

**Louise Niemer, RN, BSN, MSN, PhD, CPNP,
ARNP**
Associate Professor, Nursing
Northern Kentucky University
Highland Heights, Kentucky
Case study for Chapter 6. Assessing Nutrition
Case study for Chapter 23. Assessing the Toddler
and Preschooler

Sandra G. Raymer Raff, RN, MS, FNP
Perinatal Educator
Natividad Medical Center
Salinas, California
Case study for Chapter 20. Putting It All
Together

Joanne L. Thanavaro, RN, MSN, ARNP, BC
Assistant Professor of Nursing
Jewish Hospital College of Nursing and Allied
Health at Washington University
St. Louis, Missouri
Private Practice: Clayton Medical Consultants, Inc.
St. Louis, Missouri
Case study for Chapter 13. Assessing Peripheral-
Vascular and Lymphatic Systems

Contents

Chapter 1

Health Assessment and the Nurse

| Name: _____ | Date: _____ |
| Course: _____ | Instructor: _____ |

1. Identify the following data as subjective or objective. *Remember:* Subjective data are the client's perceptions or feelings; objective data are observable and measurable.

- Nausea _____

- Cyanosis _____

- Jaundice _____

- Edema _____

- Numbness _____

- Diaphoresis _____

- Pallor _____

- Ptosis _____

- Dizziness _____

- Stridor _____

- Palpitations _____

- Irregular pulse _____

- Shortness of breath _____

- Chest pain _____

2. Phyllis Johnson brings her 2-year-old daughter Lauren to the emergency department (ED) with a fever of 103°F. Mrs. Johnson states that Lauren has had a cough and runny nose for the past 2 days and is not sleeping or eating well. Lauren is irritable, tugs at her ear, and says "my ear hurts." Lauren's old records show that she has been treated three times over the past year for otitis media. From the data given, identify the following:

   a. Primary data source _____

   b. Secondary data source _____

   c. Subjective data _____

   d. Objective data _____

3. Match the verbal response in the first column to the appropriate communication technique in the second column.

Verbal Response	**Communication Technique**
1. "Go on."	a. Sequencing
2. "Let me see if I have this right."	b. Redirecting
3. "What does it feel like?"	c. Affirmation/facilitation
4. "You say you're afraid..."	d. Identifying themes
5. "Getting back to why you're here…"	e. Presenting reality
6. "From everything that you've said, it seems that you're concerned about…"	f. Clarifying
7. "The pain started, and then what happened?"	g. General opening
8. "Remember, you're in the hospital."	h. Reflection

4. If your client made the following statements, how would you respond?

   a. "Nurse, I have chest pain."

   _____

   b. "I'm so afraid to have surgery."

   _____

   c. "Nurse, am I going to die?"

   _____

   d. "Nurse, is it cancer?"

   _____

   e. "The night nurse made me wait all night to get pain medication."

   _____

5. The following questions/statements are common communication pitfalls. Identify the communication problem, then restate the question/statement correctly.

   a. "Does the pain go down your arm?"

   PITFALL : LEADING QUESTION ANSWER.

   DOES THE PAIN MOVE , IF SO WHERE.

b. "In my opinion, you should…"

PITFALL : GIVING ADVICE

HERE ARE SOME OPTIONS ....

c. "Don't worry, everything will be okay."

PITFALL : FALSE REASURANCE

You SEEM CONCERNED WOULD YOU LIKE TO TALK ABOUT IT

d. "You're scheduled for a laparoscopic oophorectomy."

MEDICAL JARGON

You WILL BE HAVING YOUR OVERY REMOVED SURGICALLY

e. "Things always look brighter in the morning."

USING CLICHÉ

WOULD YOU LIKE TO TALK ABOUT IT.

f. "Who brought you to the hospital? And what seems to be the problem?"

PERSISTENT & TWO MANY QUESTIONS

WHAT SEEMS TO BE THE PROBLEM

g. "Don't take it out on me!" (Response to client who says, "I can't believe I had to wait so long. This hospital is terrible!")

TAKING THINGS LITERALY

IM SORRY YOU HAD TO WAIT SO LONG

h. "Don't worry. Now let's talk about surgery." (Response to client who says, "Do you think I have cancer?")

CHANGING THE SUBJECT

WOULD TALK ABOUT THIS

i. "With your background, I'm sure you understand this." (Response to client who has a Ph.D. in chemistry and is scheduled for surgery.)

JUMPING TO CONCLUSION

LET ME EXPLAIN THE PROCEDURES OF THE SURGERY

j. "Maybe you should talk to your doctor. Now, let's talk about your diabetes." (Response to client who says, "I'm really having trouble performing sexually.")

FEELING UNCOMPFORTABLE

WOULD YOU LIKE TO TALK ABOUT THIS

k. "What's wrong with you? If you don't take your medications, you could die." (Response to client who doesn't take prescribed postoperative medications.)

ASSUMING RATHER THAN CLARYIFING

IS THERE A PROBLEM WITH TAKING YOU MEDICATIONS

6. Rose Montefalco, age 78, comes to the ED with chest pain. Subjective and objective data include the following: Client states, "My chest is killing me; it feels like I'm in a vice." Pain severity 10/10; difficulty breathing; blood pressure (BP) 170/110 mm Hg; pulse 118 beats/min and regular;

respirations 32/min; temperature 99.8°F; pulse oximetry 90% on room air; client diaphoretic, pale, and clammy; cardiac monitor shows sinus tachycardia with occasional premature ventricular contractions; electrocardiogram (ECG), chest x-ray, and cardiac enzymes done; oxygen via nasal cannula at 3 L/min. Intravenous nitroglycerin started, and chest pain decreased to 8/10 within 0.5 hour after starting nitroglycerin; BP 160/100 mm Hg; pulse 110 beats/min; respirations 28/min; pulse oximetry 93% on 3 L of oxygen. Old records show history of hypertension (HTN). From the data given, identify:

a. Primary data source _____

b. Secondary data source _____

c. Subjective data

_____

_____

d. Objective data

_____

_____

7. Document the data from question 6 using the SOAPIE method.

_____

_____

8. Document the data from question 6 using the DAR method.   DATA: MY CHEST IS KILLING ME!"
PAIN SEVERE; BP 170/110
PULSE REG, 32 RES/MIN, TEMP 9
ACTION: X-RAY, CARDIA ENZYMES, GIVE OXYGEN, & NITROGLYCERIN.
R- CHEST PAIN↓; BP 160/100 PULSE 110/MIN, RESP 28/MIN AFTER .5

9. Document the data from question 6 using the PIE method.

_____

_____

10. What's wrong with the following documentation?

  • Mrs. Kowet, age 50

  • Past health history: Normal childhood illnesses; usual immunizations

  • Review of systems: Unremarkable

  • Psychosocial profile: Social drinker, smokes occasionally

_____

11. Prioritize the following problems as 1, life-threatening; 2, urgent; and 3, can wait:

- BP 60/40 mm Hg _____

- Breathing difficulty, pulse oximetry 88% on room air _____

- Hunger and thirst _____

- Anxiety _____

- Temperature 103°F _____

Chapter 2
The Health History

1. What section of the health history contains the following data?

   a. Address _____

   b. Contact _____

   c. Genetically linked problems _____

   d. Chief complaint _____

   e. Health insurance _____

   f. Sleep and rest patterns _____

   g. Immunizations _____

   h. Exercise patterns _____

   i. Menarche, last menstrual period (LMP) _____

   j. Hospitalizations _____

   k. Breast self-examination (BSE), breast masses _____

   l. Childhood illnesses _____

   m. Symptom analysis _____

   n. Recreation/hobbies _____

   o. Testicular self-examination (TSE) and prostate examination ___

   p. Birth date _____

   q. Bowel habits and laxative use _____

   r Marital status _____

   s. Nutritional patterns _____

   t. General health _____

   u. Roles and relationships _____

   v. Glasses, last eye examination _____

   w. Religion _____

   x. Drug and alcohol use _____

   y. Last chest-x-ray, purified protein derivative (PPD)

_____

2. Match the developmental theorist in the first column to the description of his theory in the second column.

Theorist	Theory
1. Freud	a. Moral development of individual
2. Kohlberg	b. Cognitive development of individual
3. Piaget	c. Psychosocial development of individual
4. Erikson	d. Family development
5. Maslow	e. Psychosexual development of individual
6. Butler	f. Relationship between activity and aging
7. Havighurst	g. Needs as basic to self-actualization
8. Duval	h. The elderly and life review

3. You can document family history by listing or by drawing a genogram. Document your family history as a genogram.

Chapter 3

Approach to the Physical Assessment

Name: _JOHANNA EWALD_   Date: _9/13_

Course: _____   Instructor: _____

1. Match the piece of equipment in the first column to its use in the second column.

    Equipment

    1. Rectal thermometer _(D)_
    2. Bell portion of stethoscope _(E)_
    3. Diaphragm portion of stethoscope _(A)_
    4. Doppler _(B)_
    5. Snellen eye chart _(C)_
    6. Small white light of ophthalmoscope _(K)_
    7. Transilluminator _(J)_
    8. Tuning fork _(L)_
    9. Triceps skinfold calipers _(F)_
    10. Test tubes _(H)_
    11. Hammer _(I)_
    12. Goniometer _(G)_

    Use

    a. Best for detecting high-pitched sounds
    b. Detects fetal heart sounds
    c. Used to test far vision
    d. Most accurate means to obtain body temperature
    e. Best for detecting low-pitched sounds
    f. Used to measure body fat
    g. Used to measure angle of joint
    h. Used to test temperature sensation
    i. Used to test deep tendon reflexes
    j. Used to visualize fontanels and sinuses
    k. Used to assess undilated eye
    l. Used to assess vibratory sensations and hearing

2. Identify the appropriate assessment technique for the following assessment findings.

    a. Organomegaly _BI MANUAL PALPATION_
    b. Poor skin turgor _PALPATATION_
    c. Resonance _PERCUSSION SOUNDS_
    d. Skin color changes _INSPECTION_

9

e. S_1 and S_2 _AUSCULATION_

f. Skin texture _PALPATATION_

g. Fetal position _LIGHT PALPATATION_

h. Floating knee cap _PALPATION (BALLOTTEMENT)_

i. Kidney tenderness _PALPATION_

j. Deep tendon reflexes _PERCUSSION_

k. Bruit _AUSCULATATION_

l. Thrill _PALPATION_

3. Identify the part of the hand that is best for detecting the following findings:

a. Vibrations _BALL OF HAND ON THE PALM & ULNAR SURFACE_

b. Temperature _DORSAL ASPECT_

c. Pulsations _THE FINGER TIPS_

4. You are assessing Barbara La Bar, age 70, who weighs 110 lb, and her husband, Leo, age 72, who weighs 250 lb. They both have normal breath sounds, but Mrs. La Bar's are louder than her husband's, which are soft and seem diminished. How would you explain the difference?

_____

_____

5. How should you adapt your physical assessment approach for the following age groups: infants, preschoolers, adolescents, pregnant clients, and older adults?

OLDER ADULTS - NORMAL CHANGES THAT OCCUR W/AGE, DECREASE FUNCTION, &
SIGNS OF AFFECT, PREGNANT - GENERAL APPEARANCE = GENSTATIONAL AGE,
SWELLING, AFFECT & RESPONSE TO PREGNANCY. CHILD - BEHAVIOR =
DEVELOP LEVEL RELATIONSHIP WITH PARENTS. INFANTS

6. You use different positions to assess various structures. Identify the appropriate position(s) for the following examinations:

a. Pelvic examination _____

b. Prostate examination _____

c. Abdominal examination _____

d. Spinal examination _____

e. Respiratory examination _____

f. Cardiac examination _____

g. Rectal examination _____

7. Various factors can affect accurate BP readings. Identify if the BP reading would be falsely high or low for each statement.
   a. Cuff too small _FALSE HIGH READING_
   b. Cuff too loose _FALSE HIGH READING_
   c. Cuff too big _FALSE LOW READING_
   d. Arm elevated above heart level _FALSE LOW READING_
   e. Arm muscle contracted _FALSE HIGH READING_

8. Usually, either arm may be used to obtain a BP reading. Name four occasions when the use of an arm may be contraindicated.
   ARM WITH INJURY, ARM WITH IV SITE, ARM OF PATIENT WITH MASTECTOMY, ARM WITH VASCULAR ACCESS FOR DIALYSIS

9. How would you explain the importance of scanning every system in relation to the specific system being assessed?

   _____

   _____

Chapter 4
Teaching the Client

| Name: _____ | Date: _____ |
| Course: _____ | Instructor: _____ |

1. What health history data should you use to identify your client's learning needs and to develop a teaching plan?

   _____

   _____

2. What physical assessment data can you use to identify your client's learning needs and to develop a teaching plan?

   _____

   _____

3. Maria Hernandez, age 50, is divorced and of Puerto Rican descent. She has a 25-year-old married son and an 18-year-old daughter who will be attending community college in the fall. Mrs. Hernandez owns her own home in a low-income neighborhood in an urban area. She is employed full-time and works 4 days a week in 10-hour daytime shifts driving a truck. She has employer-paid health insurance for herself but no insurance for her daughter. Mrs. Hernandez's son often drives her to and from work so that her daughter can use the family car to get to her workplace.

   Mrs. Hernandez is 5 feet tall and weighs 225 lb. She has been diagnosed with HTN and non–insulin-dependent diabetes mellitus (NIDDM). According to the rules of her job, she is required to take a 45-minute lunch break and a 10-minute rest break every 1.5 hours. Mrs. Hernandez reports that she feels under a lot of pressure to make her deliveries on time, so she usually skips her breaks and grabs lunch at the drive-through of a fast-food restaurant. She also says that she doesn't like taking her "water pill" because it interferes with work and sleep and that sometimes she forgets to take her diabetes medication. She is supposed to test her blood sugar each morning with a home glucometer, but she says she does this only on the days she is not scheduled to work.

   Today Mrs. Hernandez is complaining of lower back pain and burning and irritation on urination. Her vital signs are temperature 99°F, pulse 88 beats/min, respirations 20/min, and BP 180/100 mm Hg. Her blood glucose is 160 mg/dL. Mrs. Hernandez answers your questions, makes jokes, and tells stories during the assessment. She says she thinks that she has a urinary tract infection and needs an antibiotic so she can get back on the road. She doesn't want to lose any sick days. She says that she is saving her sick days so she can help out when her new grandchild is born next month.

From the information given, identify three areas of concern that would warrant further teaching for Mrs. Hernandez.

_____

4. Identify Mrs. Hernandez's strengths that could be useful when developing a teaching plan.

_____

5. Cluster the supporting data for the following nursing diagnoses.

   a. Ineffective management of therapeutic regimen related to knowledge deficit of diabetes mellitus and HTN (management and signs/symptoms of complications).

   _____

   _____

   b. Knowledge deficit regarding management of diabetes mellitus and HTN.

   _____

   _____

6. When developing Mrs. Hernandez's teaching plan for managing her health problems, what key area do you need to consider for the plan to be successful?

   _____

Chapter 5
Assessing Wellness

Name: _____	**Date:** _____
Course: _____	**Instructor:** _____

1. Many factors affect health behavior, including the client's supports, psychological state, and access to health care. Who might be a support for your client? How might your client's psychological state affect his or her health behaviors? What might pose a barrier to health care?

   _____

   _____

2. What are *your* strengths and weaknesses regarding health and wellness? Do a self-evaluation.

   _____

   _____

3. Sleep can be affected by many factors. How might the following factors affect sleep?

   • Exercise _____

   • Nicotine use _____

   • Caffeine use _____

   • Alcohol use _____

   • Weight _____

   • Diet _____

   • Stress _____

   • Specific medical problems _____

   _____

4. Match the client in the first column to the appropriate sleep pattern in the second column.

Client	Sleep Pattern
1. Infant	a. 9–10 h/day
2. Todder/preschooler	b. 6–8 h/day
3. School-age child	c. 20 h/day
4. Adolescent	d. 6–8 h/day in segments
5. Adult	e. 10–12 h/day with nap
6. Older adult	f. 7.5 h/day (up late, sleeps late)

5. Horace Brown, age 75, is beginning an exercise program. Calculate his maximum heart rate and the minimum and ideal heart rate for cardiopulmonary fitness. (220− age × 60–80%).

_____

6. What sources of stress are typical for the following age groups?

- Infant _____

- Toddler _____

- School-age child _____

- Adolescent _____

- Young adult _____

- Middle-aged adult _____

- Older adult _____

7. What types of injuries or health problem would you assess for the following age groups?

- Infant _____

- Preschool/school-age child _____

- Adolescent _____

- Young/middle-aged adult _____

- Older adult _____

Chapter 6
Assessing Nutrition

Name: _____   Date: _____

Course: _____   Instructor: _____

1. Match the nutrient in the first column with its description in the second column.

   Nutrient

   1. Carbohydrate
   2. Proteins
   3. Fats
   4. Water
   5. High-density lipoproteins (HDLs)
   6. Low-density lipoproteins (LDLs)
   7. Vitamins

   Description

   a. Building blocks
   b. 60% of body weight
   c. Major source of energy
   d. Guard against heart disease by lowering cholesterol
   e. Provide 9 cal/g
   f. Major role in enzyme reactions
   g. Contribute to heart disease by elevating cholesterol

2. What is the difference between water-soluble and fat-soluble vitamins?

   _____

3. Identify the following vitamins as water-soluble or fat-soluble: A, B, C, D, E, and K.

   _____

4. Dietary requirements vary depending on the client's age. Name one dietary requirement and its rationale for each of the following groups.

   • Infant/toddler _____

   • Preschool child _____

   • School-age child _____

   • Adolescent _____

- Pregnant woman _____

- Older adult _____

5. Do a 24-hour recall on yourself, evaluating your diet according to the food pyramid. Note any deficits.

6. Calculate your body mass index (BMI).

7. Do a nutritional self-evaluation, using the USDA's Interactive Healthy Eating Index, available at http://147.208.9.133.

Name: _____	Date: _____
Course: _____	Instructor: _____

Abnormal Case Study: Kim Liang

Mr. Liang, age 73, immigrated to the United States from China 5 months ago to live with his 48-year-old daughter, her American husband, and their three teenage children. His daughter has been in the United States for 25 years, and she has a profitable career in international banking. Her husband is a tax attorney. Mr. Liang's daughter has brought him to her physician to be evaluated. He was treated in China for "prostate trouble," and she is concerned that his weight loss since his arrival is due to cancer.

Health History

Chief complaint:

"I'm worried that my father's weight loss is due to prostate cancer."

Symptom analysis:

P—Decreased appetite. Client eats better when daughter fixes ethnic meals.

Q—Not applicable (NA).

R—NA.

S—Weight loss of > 30 lb in past 4 to 5 months (usual weight is 175 lb); mild fatigue; denies vomiting, diarrhea, abdominal pain, dysuria, nocturia, urinary hesitancy, frequency, urgency, or dribbling/incontinence.

T—Weight loss has progressed steadily since arrival in the United States.

Current health status:

- Progressive weight loss from usual 175 lb to current weight of 145 lb over past 4 to 5 months.
- Client believes weight loss is caused by decreased intake because of lack of appetite for many American foods, but also is concerned about having cancer.

Past health history:

- Health generally "very good"; lactose intolerance since infancy; occasional cold, but never any illness that kept him from working.
- Appendectomy at age 10; corneal abrasion at age 17 incurred while playing soccer; hernia repair at age 21.
- Most significant health problem since age 21 was "prostate problem" about 3 years ago. Describes dysuria, frequency/urgency with only small amounts of urine accompanied by lower abdominal pain. Was treated with antibiotics and has had no problems since.
- Immunizations up-to-date. No additional immunizations needed to enter the United States.

Family history:

- Mother died at age 52 of breast cancer.
- Father died at age 82 of a "bad heart" (denies heart attack).
- Brother, age 78, has hypertension and glaucoma.
- Sister, age 69, alive and well.
- Grandparents died of "old age."

Review of systems:

- *General health status:* Increased fatigue over past few months.

- *Integumentary:* Skin drier than usual; blames on climate and water.
- *Head, eyes, ears, nose, throat (HEENT):* Wears glasses for reading since age 50.
- *Cardiovascular:* Denies problems.
- *Gastrointestinal:* Lactose intolerance; avoids dairy foods and uses soy-based products; daily bowel movement, brown and soft, no bleeding.
- *Genitourinary:* Denies problems; voids about four times per day, yellow urine concentrated.
- *Musculoskeletal:* Because of recent fatigue is less tolerant of physical activity (grass raking, walking).
- *Neurological:* Denies problems.
- *Lymphatic:* Occasional colds, but has not been ill or had cold since arrival in the United States; has gotten yearly flu shot since age 60.

Psychosocial profile:

- *Self-care activities:* Capable of full self-care, although daughter does his cooking and laundry.
- *Activity/exercise patterns:* Reads, visits museums, recently joined social group for Chinese-Americans, plays cards, "talks," goes to movies, enjoys helping with yard work.
- *Nutritional patterns:* Eats three meals a day. *24 hour recall:* Breakfast—8 oz. orange juice, 1 rice cake, tea. Lunch—1 cup rice with steamed broccoli, tea. Dinner—1 cup reheated rice, $^1/_4$ cup diced chicken, $^1/_2$ cup orange sherbet, tea. Family had fried chicken (he diced some breast meat for his rice), mashed potatoes, rolls, broccoli casserole, and chocolate pie for dessert. Claims this is typical intake since being in the United States. Daughter plans meals and prepares them half the time; other family members prepare remaining meals. Some ethnic foods, but household diet is predominantly "American." Lactose intolerant—develops gas/bloating; no other food intolerances/allergies.
- *Sleep/rest patterns:* Had trouble sleeping for about 2 weeks when first arrived in the United States because of time change, but no problems at present; bedroom is removed from noise and disturbance; sleeps without awakening from about 10 p.m. to 5:30 to 6:00 a.m.; feels rested.
- *Personal habits:* Smoked for about 10 years as young adult (quit for health reasons); occasionally has plum wine on special occasions; occasional beer when in China, none in the United States.
- *Occupational health patterns:* Retired chemical engineer with "good pension."
- *Environmental health patterns:* Family lives in affluent neighborhood; large, new, two-story home with five bedrooms. Client feels very safe.
- *Roles/relationships:* Wife died 11 years ago; has three children (son and daughter in United States, another son in England); close to daughter with whom he lives; immigrated here at children's urging. Likes son-in-law, thinks grandsons are spoiled but is very fond and proud of them. Interacts about once weekly with small group of Chinese-Americans (mostly men) but prefers spending time with family. Grandsons willingly take him places and spend time with him at movies, museums, and shopping.
- *Stress/coping:* Denies much stress except when grandsons argue among themselves or with parents; uses meditation and drinks tea to relax; finds yard work especially relaxing and has assumed much responsibility for this.

8. Based on his history information, should you be concerned that Mr. Liang's weight loss is related to prostate problems? What do you suspect is the cause of his weight loss?

_____

9. Evaluate Mr. Liang's diet according to the food pyramid. Are there any deficits? What are they?

_____

10. Aside from the possibility of prostate cancer, what else may account for Mr. Liang's increasing fatigue?

_____

Physical Assessment

- *General appearance:* Asian man, alert, attentive to questions, interacts politely and appropriately.
- *Vital signs:* Temperature 98.6°F; pulse 99 beats/min; respirations 20/min; BP 102/60 mm Hg; weight 147 lb; height 5 feet, 7 inches.
- *Integumentary:* Skin warm and dry with mild flaking.
- *HEENT:*
- *Head:* Normocephalic with fine, evenly distributed hair; scalp dry/flaky.
- *Eyes:* Pupils equal, responsive to light; light reflexes equal; follows object through all fields; sclerae white, conjunctivae pale.
- *Ears:* Tympanic membranes pearly gray, normal light reflex, normal mobility.
- *Nose:* Midline, no septal deviation, membranes pale/moist.
- *Mouth/throat:* Dentition intact and in good repair; tongue midline, gag intact; throat pink without exudate/erythema.

- *Neck:* No lymphadenopathy.
- *Respiratory:* Unlabored, breath sounds equal bilaterally, clear to auscultation.
- *Cardiovascular:* No visible precordial activity; point of maximal impulse not visible, palpable on midclavicular line in fifth intercostal space; normal sinus rhythm with grade 2/6 systolic murmur.
- *Gastrointestinal:* Bowel sounds present and regular, although slightly diminished; no signs of distress with palpation; no palpable masses.
- *Genitourinary:* Normal male genitalia.
- *Musculoskeletal:* Minimal muscle resistance +4/5 upper and lower extremities; full passive range of motion (ROM); extremities symmetrical, no joint swelling/inflammation.
- *Neurological:* Cranial nerves intact; deep tendon reflexes equal, +2 throughout.
- *Hematological:* Hematocrit 38, hemoglobin 13.0.

11. Because the client's daughter is concerned about the possibility of prostate cancer, what additional assessment is warranted?

_____

12. Aside from weight loss and fatigue, what additional findings would you expect if Mr. Liang did have prostate cancer?

_____

13. Mr. Liang's nutritional deficits could also result in anemia. What assessment findings suggest anemia?

_____

14. Calculate (approximately) Mr. Liang's percent of weight change and BMI. Interpret the meaning of the values obtained.

_____

15. Cluster the supporting data for the following nursing diagnoses.
    a. Nutritional imbalance, less than body requirements.

_____

_____

    b. Fluid volume deficit related to decreased oral intake.

_____

_____

c. Fatigue related to nutritional deficits.

_____

_____

16. Identify any additional nursing diagnoses for Mr. Liang.

_____

_____

Chapter 7
Spiritual Assessment

Name: _____	**Date:** _____
Course: _____	**Instructor:** _____

1. When assessing spirituality, focus on your client's behavior, communication, relationships, and environment. Identify spirituality assessment data for each of the following four areas:

   • Behavior _____

   • Communication _____

   • Relationships _____

   • Environment _____

2. Name six health care areas that might be influenced by your client's spirituality or religious beliefs.

   _____

   _____

3. How might being Jewish affect one's health practices?

   _____

4. How might being Catholic affect one's health practices?

   _____

5. How might being Islamic affect one's health practices?

   _____

6. How might being Hindu affect one's health practices?

   _____

7. How might being of the New Age faith affect one's health practices?

   _____

Name: _____		*Date:* _____	
Course: _____		*Instructor:* _____	

Abnormal Case Study: Concetta Ramirez

Mrs. Ramirez is 38-year-old Roman Catholic of Mexican descent. She is being seen by the community health nurse for follow-up after a hospitalization for cervical cancer. Mrs. Ramirez had symptoms related to her cancer for several months before seeking medical care. Her family consults a healer known as a *curandero (male)* or *curandera (female)* for most illnesses. The curandero views illness from a religious/spiritual and social context, rather than from the Western medical-scientific perspective.

Although she has received nutrition counseling, Mrs. Ramirez will not eat the foods the nurse tells her are important to aid in healing. Mrs. Ramirez states, "I got sick because I sinned. It is right that I suffer."

Health History

Biographical data:

- 38 year-old, married woman, mother of four children, ages 4, 7, 15, and 17.
- Married for 20 years. Husband Carlo works for the city as a maintenance supervisor.
- Born in El Paso, Texas, of immigrant Mexican parents.
- Moved to Philadelphia with husband 12 years ago.
- Has health insurance through husband's employment.

Current health status:

- Recently had surgery for cervical cancer.
- Scheduled for follow-up radiation therapy to begin 6 weeks after surgery.
- Tired most of the time and has difficulty completing household tasks.

Past health history:

- Gravida 5, para 4 (one stillbirth).
- Hospitalized for burns of lower legs 5 years ago after a cooking pot spilled from the stove.

Psychosocial profile:

- *Typical day:* Arises at 6 a.m., makes breakfast for husband, packs his lunch. Gets children up for school, makes breakfast, packs lunches for them. After three older children leave, has cup of coffee, makes beds, washes dishes, and straightens house. Lately needs to rest frequently as she works. Older children have been helping with younger ones. Client finds it hard to keep up with Ramon, the 4-year-old.
- *Activity/exercise patterns:* Client tries to lie down during the day but finds it difficult because of Ramon. Climbing the stairs in their three-story row home is all the exercise she can tolerate.

Spiritual Assessment

Nonverbal:

- When nurse makes home visit, client rarely speaks unless questioned.
- Client appears anxious, pacing the floor and wringing her hands.

Verbal:

- Client acknowledges that her illness is God's punishment for a sin.

- Speaks of stillbirth of her middle child, who would be 12 years old now, as another punishment.

Roles/relationships:

- Speaks of love for her husband and the strength she takes from him.
- Many family pictures in living room.
- Shows concern for her children's future and is proud of their accomplishments in school.

Environment:

- Crucifix over each doorway in home.
- Small shrine of Blessed Virgin Mary in a sheltered place in tiny front yard.
- Client fingers rosary beads during home visit.

Additional questions/answers:

- Who are your support people? "My family gives me strength to go on. I don't know what I would do without them."
- Besides your family, do you have any other support? "After I attend Mass I feel better and able to face life. Father Angelo helps me."
- What gives your life meaning? "Being able to cook and keep a clean house for my family. Being a good parent to my children and a good wife for Carlo."
- How has that changed since you became sick? "It is harder to keep up with the cooking and cleaning. The older girls help, but I want them to do good in school. It's hard to be a good mother to them in this neighborhood. There are so many temptations."

8. What religious/spiritual concerns of Mrs. Ramirez's should you be aware of?

_____

_____

9. What cultural concerns should you be aware of?

_____

_____

10. What spiritual needs does Mrs. Ramirez have?

_____

_____

Name: _____ Date: _____

Course: _____ Instructor: _____

Student Lab Sheet: Assessment of the Integumentary System

Health History

Biographical data:

Current health status: symptom analysis (PQRST)

- Changes in moles or other lesions
- Nonhealing sore or chronic ulceration
- Pruritus/itching
- Rashes
- Hair changes
- Nail changes

Past health history:

- Childhood illnesses
- Hospitalizations
- Surgeries
- Serious injuries/chronic illness
- Immunizations
- Allergies (food, drugs, and environmental)
- Medications (prescribed and OTC)
- Recent travel/military service
- Immunizations

Family history:

Review of systems:

- General health status
- HEENT
- Respiratory
- Cardiovascular
- Gastrointestinal
- Genitourinary
- Musculoskeletal
- Neurological
- Endocrine

- Lymphatic/hematological

Psychosocial profile:

- Health practices and beliefs/self-care activities
- Typical day
- Nutritional patterns (24-hour recall)
- Activity/exercise patterns
- Recreation, pets, hobbies
- Sleep/rest patterns
- Personal habits (tobacco, alcohol, caffeine, drugs)
- Occupational health patterns
- Socioeconomic status
- Environmental health patterns
- Roles, relationships, self-concept
- Cultural/religious influences
- Family roles and relationships
- Sexuality patterns
- Social supports
- Stress/coping

Physical Assessment

General survey:

- Vital signs
- Height
- Weight

Head-to-toe scan:

- HEENT
- Respiratory
- Cardiovascular
- Abdomen
- Genitourinary
- Musculoskeletal
- Neurological

Assessment of the Integumentary System

Area/Physical Assessment Skill	Assessment	Normal Findings Developmental/Cultural Variations	Student's Findings
Inspection	**Compare side to side throughout exam**		
Skin	Note color, odor, integrity	Uniform skin color with slightly darker exposed areas. No jaundice, cyanosis, pallor, erythema, hyper/hypopigmentation	
	Differentiate central (mouth and conjunctiva) cyanosis from peripheral (extremities) cyanosis	Ethnic/racial differences account for many variations in color	
	Cold or hot weather can affect surface characteristics of skin and nails	Mucous membranes and conjunctiva pink	
	In dark-skinned clients, look for color changes in conjunctiva or oral mucosa	No unusual odors	
	Identify any primary, secondary, or vascular lesions	Skin intact, no suspicious lesions	
	Describe morphology, distribution, pattern, location		
	Assess for malignant lesions		
	A = asymmetry		
	B = border irregularity		
	C = color variation		
	D = diameter > 0.5 cm		

Hair and scalp	Note color, quantity, distribution of hair, condition of scalp, presence of lesions or pediculosis **Gender, genetics, and age affect hair distribution** **Puberty marks onset of pubic hair growth with increased hair growth on legs and axillae**	Hair evenly distributed over scalp, no alopecia Normal balding patterns common to men and elderly Hair color appropriate; thins and grays with age Fine body hair (vellus) noted over most of body No lesions or pediculosis
Nails	Note color, condition, angle of attachment, presence of focal or generalized abnormalities (e.g., ridges, clubbing)	Color varies from pink to light brown in darker-skinned clients Nails well groomed and convex. Cuticle pink and intact Angle of attachment 160 degrees
Palpation	**Maintain universal precautions** **Wear gloves if assessing an open area**	
Skin	Temperature **(use dorsal part of hand)** Turgor **(test unexposed area, e.g., below clavicle)** Texture, hydration **(exposed areas tend to be drier)**	Skin warm and dry. Moisture depends on body area. Positive turgor, no tenting Texture varies from soft/fine to coarse/thick depending on area and client's age Skin coarser on extensor surfaces Older adult skin may be drier, coarser, thinner with decreased turgor and increase in lesions

Assessment of the Integumentry System (*Continued*)

Area/Physical Assessment Skill	Assessment	Normal Findings Developmental/Cultural Variations	Student's Findings
	Palpate for tenderness and surface characteristics of any lesions Check for pulsations and blanching of vascular lesions		
Hair	Palpate scalp for tenderness, masses and mobility Note texture of hair.	Scalp mobile, nontender Hair texture varies (fine, medium, coarse) depending on genetics and treatments (e.g., permanents)	
Nails	Texture and capillary refill	Nails smooth and firm; no ridges; adhere well to nail bed. Brisk capillary refill < 3 seconds	

Pertinent Health History Findings:

_____

_____

_____

_____

Pertinent Physical Assessment Findings:

_____

_____

_____

_____

Nursing Diagnoses (actual or potential) with Clustered Data:

_____

_____

_____

_____

Name:	Date:
Course:	Instructor:

Self-Evaluation Exercise

Integumentary System	YES	NO	NEED MORE PRACTICE
1. Applies knowledge of integumentary system anatomy and physiology in performing an integumentary system assessment			
2. Applies growth and development principles as applicable to the integumentary system			
3. Considers cultural variations as indicated when performing an integumentary assessment.			
4. Gathers all equipment necessary to perform an assessment of the integumentary system			
5. Obtains history specific to assessment of the integumentary system.			
6. Performs a physical assessment of the integumentary system, including General survey and head-to-toe scan Inspection Palpation			
7. Documents integumentary assessment findings.			
8. Identifies normal/abnormal findings.			
9. Clusters pertinent subjective/objective data.			
10. Identifies actual/potential health problems and states them as nursing diagnoses with supporting data.			

Chapter 9

Assessing the Head, Face, and Neck

Name: _Johanna Ewald_ **Date:** _9/27/05_

Course: _____ **Instructor:** _____

1. Anatomy review: Label the following mouth and neck structures.

_1_ • Upper lip

_2_ • Gingiva (gum)

_3_ • Hard palate

_4_ • Soft palate

_5_ • Glossopalatine arch

_6_ • Pharyngopalatine arch

_7_ • Palatine tonsil

_8_ • Uvula

_9_ • Posterior pharyngeal wall

_10_ • Papillae of tongue

_11_ • Lower lip

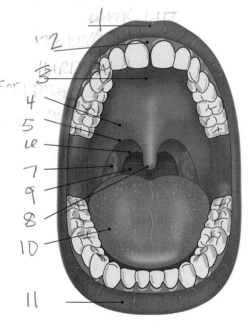

1 • Hyoid bone

2 • Thyroid cartilage

3 • Cricoid cartilage

4 • Isthmus

5 • Right thyroid lobe

7 • Left thyroid lobe

6 • Trachea

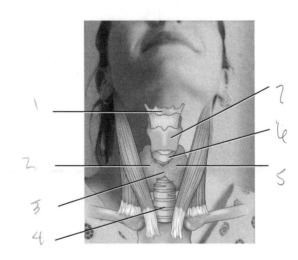

1 • Occipital

2 • Posterior auricular

4 • Preauricular

5 • Tonsilar

6 • Submandibular

7 • Submental

8 • Superficial

9 • Deep mandibular

11 • Posterior cervical

10 • Superclavicular

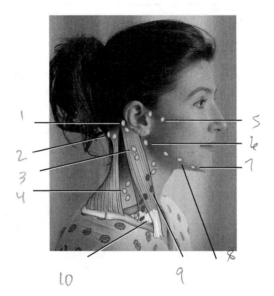

2. Match the structure in the first column to its specific function in the second column.

Structure	Function
1. Paranasal sinuses	a. Control metabolism
2. Buccal mucosa	b. Air cavities that add resonance to voice
3. Gingiva	c. Lymphatic tissue that prevents infection
4. Cilia	d. Mucous membrane of cheeks
5. Uvula	e. Drain saliva from parotid glands
6. Turbinates	f. Small hairs that filter air
7. Tonsils	g. Anchors teeth
8. Soft palate	h. Increase nasal surface area to filter, warm, and humidify air
9. Salivary glands	i. Produce saliva
10. Thyroid gland	j. Prevents food from entering nasal passages
11. Stensen's ducts	k. Drain saliva from submandibular glands
12. Wharton's ducts	l. Prevents food and saliva from entering nasopharynx

3. Mrs. Hunter says that her 4-year-old son Jared has had a sore throat and fever for 2 days and that today he complained of an earache. When inspecting Jared's throat, what three things might you expect to find?

    REDNESS OF VULVA, BUMPS ON THROAT & TONGUE, SLIMY VULVA

4. Considering Jared's age, how many teeth would you normally expect to find?

    DECIDIOUS TEETH APPOX 20

5. Name three characteristics you should note when inspecting the teeth.

    COLOR, NUMBER OF TEETH, ALIGNMENT

6. What three characteristics should you note when inspecting Jared's gums?

    COLOR, BLEEDING, RECESSION

7. Jared's rapid strep test is positive, and an antibiotic is prescribed. Considering his age, what type of antibiotic is contraindicated and why?

    TETRACYCLINE, BECAUSE IT CAUSES TEETH COLORATION

8. You also check Jared for any lymph node enlargement, and palpate tonsillar, superficial, and auricular nodes. What characteristics differentiate normal nodes from infected or malignant nodes?

    LARGE, RED, SOAK.

9. The anterior and posterior triangles are important landmarks when assessing the lymph nodes. What two muscles make up these triangles?

    TRAPEZIUS, STERNOCLEIDOMASTOID

10. You are assessing Sue Lynch, a 33-year-old woman with thyroid disease. When inspecting her thyroid gland, what three neck positions should you use?

    NEUTRAL, HYPEREXTENDED, & AS PERSON SWALLOWS

11. Landmarking is essential in palpating the thyroid gland. Where is the isthmus of the thyroid located?

    BELOW CARTILAGE

12. The thyroid gland is usually not palpable. What are the two exceptions?

    DURING PREGNANCY & PUBERTY

13. What additional assessments should you perform when assessing the head of an infant or toddler?

    PALPATATING FONTANELS & MEASURING HEAD CIRCUM

14. What two facial areas are best for assessing symmetry of facial features?

    _____

15. Although your assessment focuses on the head, face, and neck, all systems are related. What assessment findings (subjective or objective) show the relationship between the head, face, and neck and other systems?

    _____

    _____

Name: _____ Date: _____

Course: _____ Instructor: _____

Abnormal Case Study: Loretta Markus

Loretta Markus, a 65-year-old black woman, is admitted to your nursing unit after a stroke. She lives alone, and earlier today she experienced transient paralysis of her left extremities, urinary incontinence, and difficulty with her speech. After visiting the ED, she is admitted for observation and evaluation. Mrs. Markus has recovered some use of her left arm and leg, and her speech is currently intact.

Health History

Current health status:

Believes that she has been in "pretty good health." Says that she has been independent, able to care for herself, and able to perform all housework and yard work since her husband of 26 years died 2 years ago.

Past health history:

- Has had HTN for at least 10 years. Has been out of medication for some time and has not had her BP checked recently.
- Has been hospitalized only for two uncomplicated vaginal deliveries at ages 23 and 25.
- Has allergy to penicillin, which causes a generalized rash.
- Has no history of disorders involving the head, face, or neck, including hay fever, temporomandibular joint (TMJ) disorder, sinusitis, lymphoma, or thyroid disease.
- Uncertain about her immunization history, but is sure she has had no immunizations since she was quite young.
- Does not currently take any medications, but used to take hydrochlorothiazide, 25 mg daily, and propranolol, 80 mg daily.
- Experienced menopause at approximately age 50 and takes no hormones.

Family history:

- Parents both died in their mid to late 60s. Mother died of a stroke, and father died after several heart attacks.
- Uncertain of cause of death for grandparents. Knows that paternal grandfather died at fairly young age after some type of accident. Other grandparents "died of old age" in their 70s or later.
- Has three siblings, all alive: sister (age 63) and two brothers (ages 64 and 68). All have trouble with their heart or blood pressure. Oldest brother was a heavy smoker for many years and had cancer of larynx and now "has no voice box."
- Two daughters are in good health and take no medication that she knows of.
- Has seven grandchildren, all in good health.

Psychosocial profile:

- *Typical day:* Gets up at 8 a.m. and usually spends day working in house or yard. Daughters live nearby, and she visits frequently with her children, grandchildren, and nieces and nephews.
- *Nutritional patterns:* Eats three fairly well-balanced meals a day: cereal or toast for breakfast, fried meat two to three times a week, vegetables twice a day, some fruit daily. Lately, appetite has increased, but she believes that she has lost about 10 lb in the past 4 to 6 weeks "without really trying."

- *Sleep/rest patterns:* Goes to bed around 10:30 p.m. and has no trouble falling asleep. Usually sleeps well, but for the past few weeks has been wakeful at night and not sleeping well.

- *Personal habits:* Used to smoke cigarettes, but quit smoking when she developed HTN. About 3 to 4 years after she quit smoking, she started chewing tobacco and uses two to three packets per week. Rarely drinks alcohol— "maybe a sip or two of wine twice a year."

- *Occupational health patterns:* Used to work in a factory where electronic equipment components were made. Quit working when plant closed 5 years ago and she was unable to find work elsewhere.

- *Socioeconomic status:* Has a small pension from husband and draws Social Security. Says she is "barely able to make ends meet." Has had no health insurance for 5 years and is happy to be 65 so that she can start using Medicare.

- *Environmental health patterns:* Owns a small, one-story, two-bedroom home. Says it has two window air conditioning units and central heating, which are adequate.

- *Stress/coping:* Believes that she deals with stress pretty well. Is active in church and has a strong faith. Admits to being a little "on edge" and irritable lately, but has not been able to identify a cause.

16. Based on the information provided by Mrs. Markus, what, if any, real or potential problems related to her head, face, and neck do you recognize?

_____

_____

Physical Assessment

- *General appearance:* Alert, oriented; appearance consistent with stated age; slightly overweight; no apparent distress.

- *Vital signs:* Temperature 97.2°F; pulse 102 beats/min; respirations 16/min, regular and unlabored; BP 186/108 mm Hg; weight 152 lb; height 5 feet, 4 inches.

- *HEENT:*

- *Head:* Normocephalic; no obvious deformities or lesions

- *Face:* Symmetry of features; slight asymmetry of movements, with motion on left side of face diminished; no deformities.

- *Sinuses:* Nontender to palpation or percussion; transillumination not performed.

- *Eyes:* Conjunctivae pink and moist; extraocular muscles intact and conjugate.

- *Ears:* Hearing grossly intact; cerumen blockage bilaterally obscures examination.

- *Nose:* Midline placement; no nasal flaring; no discharge; mucosa pink and moist; no deformities, lesions, polyps.

- *Mouth:* Lips midline and symmetrical at rest, light brown, consistent with generalized coloring, no lesions; left weakness of lips detected with frown and exaggerated smile; full upper/lower dentures in place, removed for examination; gingiva intact, pink/moist, no erosion or lesions; 1 cm × 2 cm white patch with slight induration palpated on right buccal mucosa adjacent to right upper molars site; otherwise, buccal mucosa pink and moist with no indurations, nodules, or lesions. No visible or palpable lesions, nodules, or indurations of tongue or mucosa at floor of mouth or over palates.

- *Throat:* Tonsils not visible; uvula midline and rises with phonation; posterior wall smooth and without lesions or drainage.

- *Nodes:* Two right submandibular nodes, firm-to-hard, mobile, nontender, palpable; no other palpable nodes.

- *Thyroid:* Not visible; slightly palpable bilaterally and symmetrical; meaty consistency, no tenderness or nodules.

- *Respiratory:* Breath sounds clear bilaterally; unlabored respirations; no wheezing, crackles, or other adventitious sounds; no cough.

- *Cardiovascular:* Apical and radial pulses regular at 102 beats/min; S_1 and S_2 auscultated with no murmur, extra heart sounds; mild, 1+ edema of feet bilaterally; soft bruit bilaterally.

- *Musculoskeletal:* Full ROM; no tenderness or deformities; strength 5/5 right, 4/5 left.

- *Neurological:* Slight slurring of some words, sensation slightly diminished on left side of face, tongue strength +4/5 to the left; otherwise, cranial nerves grossly intact. Movements of right side coordinated, with +5/5 strength. Movements of left side are slightly clumsy, with +4/5 strength.

17. What factors in Mrs. Markus's assessment place her at risk for stroke?

HTNA , TIA, CARTOID BRUITIS , + FAM HISTORY, OVERWEIGHT, EATS FRIED FOOD

18. What assessment findings suggest transient ischemic attack (TIA)/stroke?

SPEECH DIFF, PARAYLISS MRINARY INCONTINENC BP 186/108

19. What factors in Mrs. Markus's assessment place her at risk for or suggest oral cancer?

POSITIVE FAMILY HISTORY, SMOKINM HISTORY, WEIGHT LOSS, LESIONS

20. Identify teaching needs for Mrs. Markus.

DELT HTN, STROKE, ORAL CANCER

21. Cluster the supporting data for the following nursing diagnoses:

a. Risk for altered nutrition less than required.

↓ MOTR FUNCTION , WEIGHT LOSS, LESIONS

b. Decreased motor function left side of face; decreased sensation.

RISK FOR ASPIRATION

c. Risk for impaired communication.

SLURREN SPEECH

22. Identify any additional nursing diagnoses for Mrs. Markus.

23. *Word jumble:* Unscramble the following words. Then unscramble the circled letters to complete the sentence: A precancerous oral lesion is called

---

   1. L U Ⓚ S L

   2. D T Ⓞ I R H Y

   3. Ⓛ V U A U

   4. E S I Ⓤ S N S

   5. Ⓘ D C O I R C

   6. O S Ⓛ T N I S

   7. E T N B Ⓐ R I U T S

   8. H Ⓟ Y L M

   9. E T Ⓔ H T

  10. I N G Ⓐ V G I

  11. C Ⓚ E N

  12. E O G T I R

Name: _____	*Date:* _____
Course: _____	*Instructor:* _____

Student Lab Sheet: Assessment of the Head, Face, and Neck

Health History

Biographical data:

Current health status: symptom analysis (PQRST):

- Headaches
- Lesions on mouth or lips
- Swelling of head or neck areas
- Difficulty chewing or swallowing
- Fatigue
- Nasal discharge or postnasal drip
- Hoarseness or voice change

Past health history:

- Childhood illnesses
- Hospitalizations
- Surgeries
- Serious injuries/chronic illness
- Immunizations
- Allergies (food, drugs, and environmental)
- Medications (prescribed and OTC)
- Recent travel/military service

Family history:

Review of systems:

- General health status
- Integumentary
- Eyes/ears
- Respiratory
- Cardiovascular
- Gastrointestinal
- Genitourinary
- Musculoskeletal
- Neurological
- Endocrine
- Lymphatic/hematological

Psychosocial profile:

- Health practices and beliefs/self-care activities
- Typical day
- Nutritional patterns (24-hour recall):
- Activity/exercise patterns
- Recreation, pets, hobbies
- Sleep/rest patterns
- Personal habits (tobacco, alcohol, caffeine, drugs)
- Occupational health patterns
- Socioeconomic status
- Environmental health patterns
- Roles, relationships, self-concept
- Cultural/religious influences
- Family roles and relationships
- Sexuality patterns
- Social supports
- Stress/coping

Physical Assessment

General survey:

- Vital signs
- Height
- Weight

Head-to-toe scan:

- General health status
- Integumentary
- Eyes/ears
- Respiratory
- Cardiovascular
- Abdomen
- Genitourinary
- Musculoskeletal
- Neurological

Assessment of the Head, Face, and Neck

HEENT (handwritten, left margin)

IN CLASS DEMO (handwritten)   *USE IN LAB* (handwritten)

Area/Physical Assessment Skill	Assessment	Normal Findings Developmental/Cultural Variations	Student's Findings
Inspection			
Head	Position: sitting		
	Note size, shape, symmetry, position	Normocephalic, erect and midline; molding in newborns from vaginal delivery	NORMOCEPHALIC, SYMMETRICAL *(handwritten)*
	Assess fontanels and measure head circumference in newborns		
Face	Note facial expression, symmetry of facial features, abnormal movements, lesions, and hair distribution	Facial expression appropriate; hair distribution appropriate for age, sex, and ethnicity; no lesions or abnormal movements	SYMMETRICAL FOLDS, *(handwritten)*
	Nasolabial folds and palpebral fissures are a good place to check for symmetry *SYMMETRY (handwritten)*	Nasolabial folds and palpebral fissures symmetrical	
Nose	Note position, deformities, septal deviation, discharge, flaring	Nose midline, symmetrical, no deviation, no flaring	SYMMETRICAL, NASAL CONGESTION / DISCHARGE *(handwritten)*
	Types of discharge: clear, bloody, purulent	Nasal mucosa pink and moist, no lesions, edema, or discharge. Septum intact.	
	If clear drainage noted from nose or ears, secondary to head trauma, suspect cerebrospinal fluid (CSF)		
	Nasal flaring sign of respiratory distress in newborns		
	Use nasoscope or otoscope with nasal speculum to assess nasal mucosa for color, intactness, lesions, edema, and discharge		

			(handwritten notes)
Frontal and maxillary sinuses	**Frontal sinuses are located above eyebrow; maxillary below eyes** Note periorbital edema or "dark circles" under eyes Transilluminate sinuses if indicated	No periorbital edema noted Sinuses clear; positive transillumination	
Parotid and submandibular glands	**Parotid glands located in front of ears; submandibular glands under mandible** Note any edema, redness	No edema or redness noted over salivary glands	NO INFLAMATION
Lips	Note color, condition, lesions, breath odor, pursed-lip breathing	Lips pink, moist, intact, no lesions, no unusual odor (halitosis), no pursed-lip breathing	NO IRREGULARITIES PINK & MOIST
Oral mucosa	Note color, conditions, lesions *Leukoplakia or "smoker's" lesion is a white, nontender, precancerous lesion that warrants follow-up* Inspect Stensen's and Wharton's ducts for inflammation **Stensen's duct located opposite second upper molar; Wharton's duct on floor of mouth under tongue**	Oral mucosa pink, moist, intact, no lesions Oral mucosa may be bluish or have patchy appearance in dark-skinned individuals Stensen's and Wharton's ducts patent; no inflammation	MOIST , PINK
Gingivae	Note color, condition, retraction, hypertrophy, edema, bleeding, lesions	Gingivae pink, moist, intact; no bleeding, edema, retraction, or lesions During pregnancy, gingivae may normally atrophy	PINK , INTACK

Assessment of the Head, Face, and Neck (*Continued*)

Area/Physical Assessment Skill	Assessment	Normal Findings Developmental/Cultural Variations	Student's Findings
Teeth	Note number, color, condition, occlusion, missing or loose teeth *A loose tooth could dislodge and obstruct the airway*	32 teeth (adult), 20 (child), white, in good repair, none missing or loose. Edges smooth, no caries. Good occlusion	
Tongue	Note color, texture, position, mobility, involuntary movements and lesions Mobility of tongue **(CN XII)**	Tongue pink, moist, papillae intact, midline with full mobility, no lesions or involuntary movements, geographic tongue normal variation	
Oropharynx, hard/soft palate, tonsils, uvula	Note color, condition, lesions, drainage, exudates, edema Using penlight, have patient say "ah" and look for symmetrical rise of uvula and swallow reflex **(CN IX and X)**	Hard and soft palate pink and intact, tonsils pink, symmetrical, +1, no lesions or exudates, symmetrical rise of uvula, positive swallow reflex	
Neck, thyroid and cervical lymph nodes	**Inspect neck in neutral position, hyperextended, and as client swallows** Note symmetry, ROM, and condition of skin. Note thyroid or lymph node enlargement **Use anterior and posterior triangles as landmarks**	Neck symmetrical, active ROM, no masses, skin intact Larynx and trachea rise with swallowing Older clients may have limited ROM of neck	

Palpation		
Maintain universal precautions. Wear gloves when palpating oral structures or if lesions suspected		
Head	Note masses, tenderness, scalp mobility. In children <2 years old, assess fontanels and measure head circumference **Anterior fontenel closes by 18–24 months; posterior fontanel by 2 months**	Head symmetrical, no masses, nontender, scalp freely movable For children: Note if head circumference is above or below growth norms for established growth percentile. Fontanels should be soft and flat
Face	Palpate bony structures of face and jaw. Note condition and symmetry, tenderness, muscle tone, and TMJ function	Facial bones smooth, intact, symmetrical, nontender. Good muscle tone TMJ with full active ROM, no crepitation or tenderness noted
Nose	Palpate for tenderness, deformity, and patency	No nasal tenderness or deformities. Nares patent
Frontal and maxilllary sinuses	Palpate for tenderness	Sinuses nontender
Parotid and submandibular glands	Parotid glands located in front of ears; submandibular glands under mandible Note enlargement or tenderness	Salivary glands not enlarged, nontender
Lips and tongue	Palpate for tenderness, muscle tone, and lesions	Soft, nontender with good muscle tone. No lesions
Oropharynx	Test gag reflex by touching back of soft palate with tongue blade *Absent gag reflex poses risk for aspiration*	Positive gag reflex (CN IX and X)

Assessment of the Head, Face, and Neck (Continued)

Area/Physical Assessment Skill	Assessment	Normal Findings Developmental/Cultural Variations	Student's Findings
Thyroid gland	Use anterior or posterior approach	Nonpalpable, nontender thyroid	
	Locate thyroid isthmus below cricoid cartilage. Palpate at edge of sternocleidomastoid as client swallows	Small, smooth edge of thyroid may be palpable. Palpable in high-output states such as pregnancy and puberty; not normally palpable in elderly	
Cervical lymph nodes	Note size, shape, consistency, tenderness, and nodules	Nonpalpable, nontender cervical lymph nodes	
	Note size, shape, symmetry, consistency, mobility, tenderness, and temperature of palpable nodes	Superficial nodes or "shotty" node may be palpable, small <1 cm, mobile, soft-to-firm, nontender	
	Use light palpation with your finger pads in a circular movement	May normally be palpable in children; normal node <3 cm, firm, round, well-defined, mobile, nontender, symmetrical	
Percussion	**Use direct percussion**		
Frontal and maxillary sinuses	Percuss sinuses for tenderness	Sinuses nontender	
Auscultation	**Use bell of stethoscope**		
Thyroid gland	If thyroid gland enlarged, auscultate for bruits while client holds breath	No bruits	

Pertinent Health History Findings:

Pertinent Physical Assessment Findings:

Nursing Diagnoses (actual or potential) with Clustered Data:

Name: _____	*Date:* _____
Course: _____	*Instructor:* _____

Self-Evaluation Exercise

Head, Face, and Neck	YES	NO	NEED MORE PRACTICE
1. Applies knowledge of head, face, and neck anatomy and physiology in performing head, face, and neck assessment			
2. Applies growth and development principles as applicable to the head, face, and neck regions			
3. Considers cultural variations as indicated when performing a head, face, and neck assessment			
4. Gathers all equipment necessary to perform a head, face, and neck assessment			
5. Obtains history specific to a head, face, and neck assessment			
6. Performs a physical assessment of the head, face, and neck, including • General survey and head-to-toe scan • Inspection • Palpation • Percussion • Auscultation			
7. Documents head, face, and neck assessment findings			
8. Identifies normal/abnormal findings			
9. Clusters pertinent subjective/objective data			
10. Identifies actual/potential health problems and states them as nursing diagnoses with supporting data			

Chapter 10

Assessing the Eye and Ear

Name: _____   Date: _____

Course: _____   Instructor: _____

Eye

1. Anatomy review: Label the following eye structures:

- Eyebrow

- Upper eyelid

- Iris

- Pupil

- Caruncle

- Lower eyelid

- Eyelash

- Sclera covered by bulbar conjunctiva

- Palpebral conjunctiva covers lids

- Lacrimal punctum

- Medial canthus

- Lateral canthus

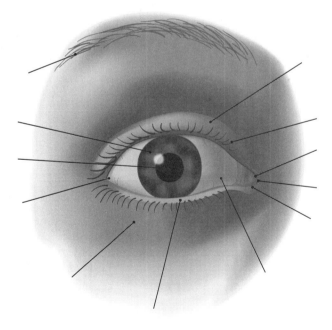

- Cornea

- Anterior chamber

- Orbicularis oculi muscle

- Iris

- Pupil

- Tarsal plate

- Meibomian gland in tarsal plate

- Orbital fat

- Lens

- Sclera

- Posterior chamber

- Ciliary body

- Frontal bone

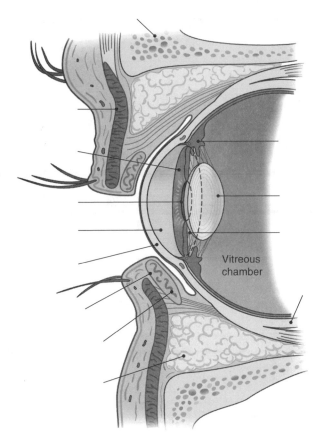

- Optic disc

- Physiologic cup

- Macula

- Fovea centralis

- Artery

- Vein

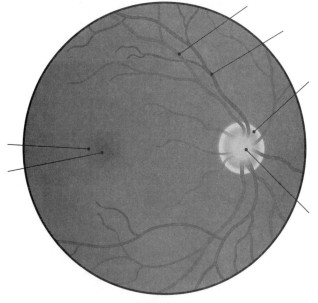

Right eye

2. Match the structure in the first column to its specific function in the second column.

Structure	Function
1. Bulbar conjunctiva	a. Drain for aqueous humor; helps control intraocular pressure
2. Cornea	b. Area of central vision
3. Lens	c. Area where optic nerve enters eye
4. Iris	d. Biconvex disk through which light and images pass
5. Palpebral conjunctiva	e. Colored, circular muscular diaphragm
6. Sclera	f. Mucous membrane that lines eyeball
7. Lacrimal gland	g. Clear, jelly-like substance that cushions retina and helps maintain eye shape
8. Macula	h. Area between cornea and iris
9. Optic disk	i. Area between iris and lens
10. Anterior chamber	j. White, tough avascular layer that gives eye structure and shape
11. Canal of Schlemm	k. Produces tears
12. Posterior chamber	l. Clear fluid that supplies lens and cornea with nutrition
13. Vitreous humor	m. Mucous membrane that lines eyelids
14. Aqueous humor	n. Outer layer of eye; avascular and transparent

3. Dan Jordan, a 55-year-old man with type 2 diabetes, is here for his annual eye examination. When you measure his visual acuity, the results are OD 20/50, OS 20/40, OU 20/40. Mr. Jordan asks you, "What does this mean?" How would you explain these results to him?

_____

_____

4. Normal far vision for an adult is 20/20. Would you expect a toddler to have 20/20 vision?

_____

_____

5. Name three tests used to measure the extraocular muscles.

_____

6. Match the structure in the first column with possible abnormal assessment findings in the second column.

Structure	Abnormal Findings
1. Lids	a. Ectropion
2. Lashes	b. Arcus senilis
3. Cornea	c. Xanthelasma
4. Bulbar conjunctiva	d. Cataract
5. Lens	e. "Pink eye"
6. Anterior chamber	f. Jaundice
7. Sclera	g. Increased intraocular pressure

7. You are performing a funduscopic examination on Mr. Jordan. Identify three key details to remember when using an ophthalmoscope.

_____

_____

8. Describe the function of the different light apertures of the ophthalmoscope.

   a. Small white light _____

   b. Large white light _____

   c. Blue light _____

   d. Green light _____

   e. Grid _____

   f. Slit of white light _____

9. Although your assessment focuses on the eyes, all systems are related. What assessment findings (subjective or objective) show the relationship between the eyes and other systems?

_____

_____

Name: _____	*Date:* _____
Course: _____	*Instructor:* _____

Abnormal Case Study: Brenda Williams

Brenda Williams is a 45-year-old, married black woman and mother of two. A part-time computer analyst, she presents in the ED with complaints of severe eye pain. Because this is an acute problem, you do a focused assessment. Findings suggest primary angle-closure glaucoma.

Health History

Chief complaint:

"I have terrible eye pain."

Symptom analysis:

P—No precipitating factor and nothing seems to make it better.

Q—"Feels like someone is stabbing my eye."

R—Colored halos around lights, blurred vision, nausea and vomiting.

S—10/10.

T—Acute onset.

Current health status:

- Denies history of eye problems; doesn't wear corrective lenses.

- Denies any medical problems.
- Last eye examination 2 years ago.

Physical Assessment

- *Visual acuity:* Unable to test near and far vision because of blurred vision.
- *Peripheral vision:* Field cuts noted in temporal fields.
- *Extraocular movement:* Intact.
- *External structures:* Eyes red, cornea has frosted appearance.
- *Internal structures:* Optic disk cupping

10. Considering Mrs. Williams's diagnosis of primary angle-closure glaucoma, what additional history question should you ask her? Why?

    WHAT MEDS ARE YOU TAKING? MAY CAUSE ISSUES WITH VISION

11. What additional test is indicated in view of Mrs. Williams's presenting signs and symptoms?

    TONOMETRY

12. Primary angle-closure glaucoma is considered a medical ocular emergency. What would likely result if Mrs. Williams's problem goes untreated?

    BLINDNESS

13. What factor placed Mrs. Williams at risk for glaucoma?

RACE , GLAUCOMA IN AF AMERICANS

14. Cluster the data for the following nursing diagnoses:

a. Pain related to increased intraocular pressure.

EYE PAIN

b. Risk for injury related to visual acuity deficits.

DECREASED VISION / BLURRED

c. Disturbed sensory perception (vision) related to pathological process.

BLURRED VISSION + PERHIRAL , COLOR HALOS

15. Identify any additional nursing diagnoses for Mrs. Williams.

16. *Word jumble:* Unscramble the following words. Then unscramble the circled letters to complete the sentence: Always examine the _____ last on funduscopic examination.

1. L A (C) R S E

2. R S I I

3. A L D E (M) I   C U S T H N A

4. E N R C A O

5. L R C I (L) M A A   L N D A G

6. T A I N R E

7. (A) N V T I C J N U O C

8. (U) P L I P

9. N S E L

10. E V O F (A)

Name: _____	*Date:* _____
Course: _____	*Instructor:* _____

Student Lab Sheet: Assessment of the Eyes

Health History

Biographical data:

Current health status: symptom analysis (PQRST)

- Vision loss
- Tearing
- Eye pain
- Changes in eye appearance
- Blurred vision
- Dry eyes
- Double vision
- Drainage

Past health history:

- Childhood illnesses
- Hospitalizations
- Surgeries
- Serious injuries/chronic illness
- Immunizations
- Allergies (food, drugs, environmental)
- Medications (prescribed and OTC)
- Recent travel/military service

Family history:

Review of systems:

- General health status
- HEENT
- Respiratory
- Cardiovascular
- Gastrointestinal
- Genitourinary
- Musculoskeletal
- Neurological
- Endocrine
- Lymphatic/hematological

Psychosocial profile:

- Health practices and beliefs/self-care activities
- Typical day
- Nutritional patterns (24-hour recall)
- Activity/exercise patterns
- Recreation, pets, hobbies
- Sleep/rest patterns
- Personal habits (tobacco, alcohol, caffeine, and drugs)
- Occupational health patterns
- Socioeconomic status
- Environmental health patterns
- Roles, relationships, self-concept
- Cultural/religious influences
- Family roles/relationships
- Sexuality patterns
- Social supports
- Stress/coping

Physical Assessment

General survey:

- Vital signs
- Height
- Weight

Head-to-toe scan:

- Integumentary
- Head, nose, throat
- Respiratory
- Cardiovascular
- Abdomen
- Genitourinary
- Musculoskeletal
- Neurological

1st GENERAL SURVEY:

GREET, NAME, ASK HOW THEY FEEL (FIRST?)

Assessment of the Eyes

Area/Physical Assessment Skill	Assessment	Normal Findings Developmental/Cultural Variations	Student's Findings
Visual acuity	**Measure each eye separately, then together, with and without corrective lenses** **Tests CN I**		
Far	Depending on client's age and literacy level, use Snellen eye chart, Snellen E chart, or Stycar chart Visual acuity represented by fraction with **numerator 20—number of feet client stands from chart—and denominator—number of feet someone with 20/20 vision can read chart—e.g., 20/40 vision** **No more than 2 mistakes per line**	20/20 OD, OS, OU Child's vision does not reach 20/20 until around age 6 or 7	
Near	Assess ability to read newsprint held 13–15 inches from eyes Use print-sized pictures if client unable to read	Near vision intact Presbyopia (farsightedness) commonly occurs with aging	
Color vision	Differentiate patterns of colors on color plates or identify color bars on Snellen eye chart	Color vision intact	

	Technique	Normal Findings
Peripheral vision	Assess ability to detect movement coming in from periphery (inferior, superior, temporal, and nasal fields) ***Sudden loss of peripheral vision may be a sign of acute glaucoma, a medical emergency. Needs immediate ophthalmology referral***	Peripheral vision intact OU, all fields
Extraocular muscles	Inspect eyes for parallel alignment and corneal light reflex **(look for the sparkle in eyes)** Put eyes through ROM, six cardinal fields of vision **(tests CN III, IV, VI)** Perform cover-uncover test, check for drifting	Eyes in parallel alignment. Corneal light reflex symmetrical, extraocular movement intact OU, no lid lag or nystagmus. No wandering with cover-uncover test
Inspection **External eye structures**	**Position: sitting**	
General appearance	Note appearance and parallel alignment	Eyes clear and bright. Equal parallel alignment
Eyelids	Note color, lesions, edema, lid lag, and symmetry of palpebral fissures **(opening of eyes between upper and lower lids)**	Color consistent with client's complexion. No lesions or edema. Palpebral fissures symmetrical. No lid lag
Eyelashes	Note symmetry and distribution note entropion, ectropion	Eyelashes evenly distributed, no ectropion or entropion
Lacrimal ducts, puncta	Note color, edema, excessive tearing, or drainage	Puncta pale pink and patent, no excessive tearing or dryness, drainage, or edema

Assessment of the Eyes (Continued)

Area/Physical Assessment Skill	Assessment	Normal Findings Developmental/Cultural Variations	Student's Findings
Conjunctiva	Assess color, moisture, lesions, and foreign bodies **Palpebral conjunctiva covers lids; bulbar conjunctiva covers eyeball**	Conjunctiva clear, pink, and moist; no lesions Pull Down Lids	
Sclera	Note color, moisture, and lesions or tears Examine cornea from oblique angle	Sclera white and intact, no lesions or tears Brown spots, muddy sclera, may be seen in persons with dark skin	
Cornea	Note clarity, lesions, or abrasions Test corneal reflex (CN V and VII) **Instead of touching cornea with wisp of cotton, use a needleless syringe and either shoot small amount of air over cornea or gently touch lashes and look for blink reflex**	Cornea clear without opacities, lesions, or abrasions Arcus senilis (white ring around the edge of cornea) common finding in elderly Positive corneal reflex	
Anterior chamber	Inspect for clarity, bulging of iris, and blood **To inspect with client's eyes looking straight ahead, look across eye from the side**	Anterior chamber clear, no blood or bulging of iris	
Iris	Note color, size, shape, and symmetry	Irises round and symmetrical	

Pupils	Note size, shape, reaction to light (direct and consensual), and test for accommodation. **Tests CN III** **Consensual reaction: pupil not receiving light stimulus reacts same as pupil receiving stimulus** ***Changes in pupils, such as unequal or dilated, may be a sign of increased intracranial pressure***	Pupil size 3-5 mm. Normal size depends on age, larger in children, smaller in elderly. No miosis or mydriasis Pupils equal, round, reactive to light, and accommodation direct and consensual (PERRLA) Reaction to light: pupils constrict Accommodation: pupils converge and constrict Older client may have decreased accommodation Anisocoria (unequal pupils) if < 0.5 mm can be normal variation		
Palpation	**Maintain universal precautions** **Wear gloves if there is eye drainage**			
Eyeball	**Gently palpate globe with fingertips or thumb on upper lids over sclera** Note consistency and tenderness ***Do not palpate eyeball in clients with eye trauma or known glaucoma***	Eyeball firm and nontender CHECK		
Lacrimal apparatus (tear glands and ducts)	Palpate below eyebrow and inner canthus of eye. Note tenderness or excessive tearing or discharge from punctae	Lacrimal gland nontender, no drainage or excessive tearing		

Assessment of the Eyes (Continued)

Area/Physical Assessment Skill	Assessment	Normal Findings Developmental/Cultural Variations	Student's Findings
Ophthalmoscopy	**Perform in dark room. Examine same eye to same eye (your right eye to client's right eye). Use small white light for undilated pupil**		
Red reflex	Note presence, opacities **Approach from oblique angle, about 14 inches from client**	Positive red reflex, no opacities	
Optic disk and physiological cup	**Located nasally** Note size, shape, borders, color, cup:disk ratio	Optic disk round, with sharp margins; cup:disc ratio 1:2 DD. Color depends on client's pigmentation. Yellow-to-orange with white cup	
Retinal vessels	Assess size ratio of arteries and veins, color, arteriole light reflex, crossings **Arteries and veins come out of disk in pairs. Veins normally darker and larger than arteries**	Vessels noted. Arteriovenous ratio 2:3 or 4:5. Positive arteriole light reflex. Arteriovenous crossings smooth, no nicking or narrowing	
Retina	Assess color, texture, exudates, lesions, hemorrhages, or aneurysms	Color varies from pale yellow to orange-red, depending on client's pigmentation. The darker the person, the darker the background. Texture finely granular. No lesions, hemorrhages, exudates, or aneurysms	
Macula, fovea centralis	**Always examine last** Note, color, size, location, and lesions **Macula is darker area temporal to disk**	Macula darker area on retina, 2 DD temporal to OD, 1 DD in size, no lesions, and positive fovea light reflex	

Pertinent Health History Findings:

Pertinent Physical Assessment Findings:

Nursing Diagnoses (actual or potential) with Clustered Data:

Name: _____   Date: _____

Course: _____   Instructor: _____

Self-Evaluation Exercise

Eyes	YES	NO	NEED MORE PRACTICE
1. Applies knowledge of anatomy and physiology of the eye in performing an eye assessment			
2. Applies growth and development principles as applicable to the eye			
3. Considers cultural variations as indicated when performing an eye assessment			
4. Gathers all equipment necessary to perform an eye assessment			
5. Obtains history specific to assessment of the eye			
6. Performs a physical assessment of the eye, including • General survey and head-to-toe scan • Visual testing • Inspection of external structures • Palpating of external structures • Ophthalmoscopy			
7. Documents eye assessment findings			
8. Identifies normal/abnormal findings			
9. Clusters pertinent subjective/objective data			
10. Identifies actual/potential health problems and states them as nursing diagnoses with supporting data			

Name: _____ Date: _____

Course: _____ Instructor: _____

Ear

1. Anatomy review: Label the following ear structures:

- Helix

- Tragus

- Lobule

- Antitragus

- Antihelix

- External auditory canal

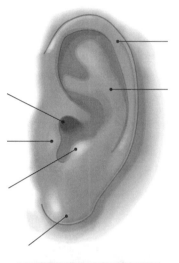

- Pars tensa

- Pars flaccida

- Cone of light

- Umbo

- Malleous

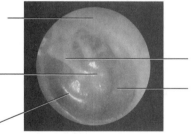

2. Match the structure in the first column to its specific function in the second column.

Structure	Function
1. Auricle	a. Light reflection on tympanic membrane
2. Tympanic membrane	b. Located in inner ear; organ of hearing that transmits sound to CN VIII
3. Cochlea	c. External ear; collects sound waves
4. Auditory ossicles	d. Eardrum
5. Cone of light	e. Tube from middle ear to nasopharynx that equalizes pressure in middle ear
6. Organ of Corti	f. Ear wax
7. Eustachian tube	g. Smallest bones of body in middle ear; transmit sound vibrations
8. Cerumen	h. Shell-like structure in inner ear that transmits sound vibrations

3. Mrs. Hudson says that her son, Jimmy, age 2, has had a fever for 2 days and started complaining of an earache today. Part of your assessment should include examining the ears. You discover that Jimmy's gross hearing is diminished. List five questions that may help you identify contributing/risk factors for hearing loss.

_____

_____

4. You perform the Weber test on Jimmy, checking for lateralization of sound. If Jimmy had a conductive hearing loss, to which ear would the sound lateralize? If he has a sensorineural hearing loss, to which ear would the sound lateralize?

_____

5. Next, you perform the Rinne test to compare bone conduction with air conduction. What would you expect the normal findings to be? What findings would you expect if Jimmy has a conductive hearing loss?

_____

_____

6. Now, inspect Jimmy's external ear and look for drainage. Name three types of drainage you might see, and describe the significance of each.

_____

_____

7. Before you perform the otoscopic examination, name three places that you need to palpate for tenderness before otoscope insertion.

_____

_____

8. To straighten a young child's ear canal, which way should the auricle be positioned? What about an adult's ear canal?

_____

9. Name three characteristics you should note when assessing the tympanic membrane.

_____

10. Jimmy's eardrum is red and bulging. Mrs. Hudson says, "Jimmy gets a lot of ear infections. Why?" How would answer this question?

_____

_____

11. Although your assessment focuses on the ears, all systems are related. What assessment findings (subjective or objective) show the relationship between the ears and other systems?

_____

_____

Name: _____	Date: _____
Course: _____	Instructor: _____

Abnormal Case Study: Brian Chapin

Mrs. Chapin brings her 3-year-old son, Brian, for treatment of recurrent earache. Brian has had frequent ear infections. He caught a cold last week and now is irritable, tugging at his ear, and not sleeping or eating well. His temperature is 101°F.

Health History

Chief complaint:

"My ear hurts."

Current health status:

- Recent upper respiratory infection.
- Mother reports irritability, tugging at ear, not sleeping or eating well.
- History of recurrent ear infections.
- No known allergies to drugs, food, or environmental factors.
- Family history of otitis media; father had frequent ear infections as a child.

Physical Assessment

- Tugging at ear and irritable.
- Temperature 101°F.
- External ear tenderness.
- External ear canal patent, no drainage.
- Tympanic membrane red and bulging, diffuse cone of light, no perforation.
- Productive cough, yellow mucus.
- Red pharynx.
- Tonsils enlarged and red without exudates.
- Lungs clear.

12. What factors put Brian at risk for otitis media?

_____

_____

13. What other history findings would identify additional risk factors for otitis media?

_____

14. Considering Brian's findings, what additional assessment of the tympanic membrane is indicated?

_____

15. Cluster the supporting data for the following nursing diagnoses:

    a. Pain related to increased fluid and pressure in the ear.

    _____

    _____

    b. Risk for disturbed sensory perception (hearing) related to pathological process.

    _____

    _____

    c. Risk for fluid volume deficit.

    _____

    _____

    d. Sleep pattern disturbance.

    _____

16. Identify any additional nursing diagnoses for Brian.

    _____

    _____

17. *Word jumble:* Unscramble the following words. Then unscramble the circled letters to complete the sentence: Another word for swimmer's ear is

    _____

    1. (T) S I O I T (E) D I M A

    2. G T U S A (R)

    3. O S T M D A (I)

    4. C S I (N) U

    5. L O L M U A S (E) L

    6. E P S (A) T S

    7. H C E A L (O) C

    8. I H (L) E (X)

    9. S (I) X (S) O E (T) I O S

    10. A L C O H M (T) E S E O A T

Name: _____	*Date:* _____
Course: _____	*Instructor:* _____

Student Lab Sheet: Assessment of the Ears

Health History

Biographical data:

Current health status: symptom analysis (PQRST):

- Hearing loss
- Vertigo
- Tinnitus
- Otorrhea
- Otalgia

Past health history:

- Childhood illnesses
- Hospitalizations
- Surgeries
- Serious injuries/chronic illness
- Immunizations
- Allergies (food, drugs, environmental)
- Medications (prescribed and OTC)
- Recent travel/military service

Family history:

Review of systems:

- General health status
- Head, nose, throat
- Respiratory
- Cardiovascular
- Gastrointestinal
- Genitourinary
- Musculoskeletal
- Neurological
- Endocrine
- Lymphatic/hematological

Psychosocial profile:

- Health practices and beliefs/self-care activities
- Typical day
- Nutritional patterns (24-hour recall)
- Activity/exercise patterns
- Recreation, pets, hobbies
- Sleep/rest patterns
- Personal habits (tobacco, alcohol, caffeine, and drugs)
- Occupational health patterns
- Socioeconomic status
- Environmental health patterns
- Roles, relationships, self-concept
- Cultural/religious influences
- Family roles/relationships
- Sexuality patterns
- Social supports
- Stress/coping

Physical Assessment

General survey:

- Vital signs
- Height
- Weight

Head-to-toe scan:

- Integumentary
- Head, nose, throat
- Respiratory
- Cardiovascular
- Abdomen
- Genitourinary
- Musculoskeletal
- Neurological

Assessment of Ears

Area/Physical Assessment Skill	Assessment	Normal Findings Developmental/Cultural Variations	Student's Findings
Inspection			
External ear	**Position: sitting; supine for infant to immobilize head**		
	Note position, shape, size, symmetry, color, lesions, and drainage (clear, bloody, or purulent). *Clear drainage from nose or ears secondary to head trauma may be CSF*	Vertical ear position with < 10 degree lateral posterior slant. Ears aligned with eyes, symmetrical, no redness, lesions, or drainage	
	Note angle of attachment (**draw imaginary line from top of helix to external canthus of eye, then a perpendicular line in front of ear)**		
Palpation	**Maintain universal precautions** **Wear gloves if drainage present**		
External ear	Assess consistency, tenderness, and lesions	Helix soft and pliable, nontender, no nodules or lesions	
	Palpate tragus and mastoid process, and pull helix forward before inserting otoscope. **Tenderness may signal ear infection, so proceed carefully**		

		Normal Findings		
Otoscopic exam	**Use largest and shortest speculum ear canal can accommodate (4, 5, or 6 mm, 0.5 inch). Have client tilt head to opposite side being examined** **Pull helix up and back for adult and down for child. Always look into canal before inserting otoscope** **Insert 0.5 inch for an adult; insert 0.25 inch for child. Avoid inner two thirds of canal, which is over temporal bone and is sensitive**			
External ear canal	Note color, drainage, patency, edema, lesions, or foreign objects **Cerumen is only normal drainage in ear**	Ear canal light colored and patent; small amount of yellow cerumen and hair; no lesions, exudates, or foreign objects Color and amount of cerumen varies depending on ethnicity		
Tympanic membrane	Note position of landmarks (cone of light, pars flaccida, pars tensa, malleus, and umbo). **Ears are mirror images, cone of light is at 7 o'clock in left ear and 5 o'clock in right ear**	Tympanic membrane pearly gray, intact, mobile, no lesions or exudates. Landmarks appropriately noted. No bulging or retraction of tympanic membrane		
	Note intactness of tympanic membrane, color, lesions, and exudates. Assess mobility of tympanic membrane in children. Use pneumatic attachment to assess mobility of tympanic membrane *Never irrigate ear canal unless you are sure tympanic membrane is intact*			

Assessment of Ears (Continued)

Area/Physical Assessment Skill	Assessment	Normal Findings Developmental/Cultural Variations	Student's Findings
Hearing	**Test each ear separately**		
Gross hearing	Whispered voice test to assess for low-pitch deficits **(1-2 feet from ear)** Ticking watch test to assess for high-pitch deficits **(5 inches from ear)**	Gross hearing intact bilaterally.	
Weber test	Place vibrating tuning fork on forehead or top of head to assess bone conduction *Do not touch prongs of tuning fork—it dampens vibration*	Negative lateralization of sound, heard equally in both ears	
Rinne test	Compare bone conduction with air conduction. Place vibrating tuning fork on mastoid (bone conduction) until no longer heard, then move fork to in front of ear (air conduction). Time how long sound is heard	Sound transmission through air is normally twice as long as sound transmission through bone AC>BC	
Balance			
Romberg test	Perform Romberg test (see Chapter 18: Assessing the Musculoskeletal System) with eyes open, then closed	Negative Romberg	

Pertinent Health History Findings:

_____
_____
_____
_____

Pertinent Physical Assessment Findings:

_____
_____
_____
_____

Nursing Diagnoses (actual or potential) with Clustered Data:

_____
_____
_____
_____

Name: _____   Date: _____

Course: _____   Instructor: _____

Self-Evaluation Exercise

Ears	YES	NO	NEED MORE PRACTICE
1. Applies knowledge of anatomy and physiology of the ear in performing an ear assessment			
2. Applies growth and development principles as applicable to the ear			
3. Considers cultural variations as indicated when performing an ear assessment			
4. Gathers all equipment necessary to perform an ear assessment			
5. Obtains history specific to assessment of the ear			
6. Performs a physical assessment of the ear, including • General survey and head-to-toe scan • Hearing testing • Inspection of external structures • Palpation of external structures • Otoscopic exam			
7. Documents ear assessment findings			
8. Identifies normal/abnormal findings			
9. Clusters pertinent subjective/objective data			
10. Identifies actual/potential health problems and states them as nursing diagnoses with supporting data			

Chapter 11

Assessing the Respiratory System

Name: _____	Date: _____
Course: _____	Instructor: _____

1. Anatomy review: Label the following structures.

   - Nasal cavity
   - Nasopharynx
   - Oropharynx
   - Laryngopharynx
   - Esophagus
   - Trachea
   - Larynx
   - Right bronchial tree
   - Left bronchial tree
   - Mediastinum
   - Parietal pleura
   - Pulmonary artery
   - Terminal bronchiole
   - Capillaries
   - Pulmonary vein
   - Alveolar duct
   - Alveolus
   - Interalveolar septum
   - Acinus

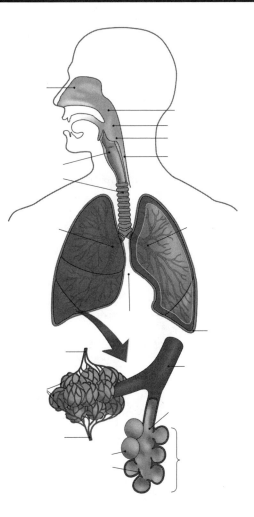

2. Match the structure in the first column to its specific function in the second column.

Structure	**Function**
1. Nasal cavity	a. Prevents food from entering trachea
2. Pleura	b. Primary muscle for breathing
3. Alveoli	c. Warms and filters air
4. Diaphragm	d. Contains vocal cords
5. Epiglottis	e. Protective lining of lung
6. Larynx	f. Functional unit of lung

3. Match the breath sound in the first column to the description in the second column.

Breath Sound	**Description**
1. Vesicular	a. Abnormal voice sound "ee" to "aa"
2. Crackles	b. High-pitched musical sound heard during acute asthmatic attack
3. Bronchial	c. Normal breath sound heard over manubrium with equal respiratory phases
4. Rhonchi	d. "Popping" sound heard predominately during inspiration; sign of congestive heart failure
5. Bronchovesicular	e. High-pitched inspiratory sound; sign of upper airway obstruction
6. Wheezes	f. Abnormal voice sound, clearer transmission of spoken voice sound
7. Egophony	g. "Rattle" sound primarily heard on expiration in upper airway resulting from secretions
8. Stridor	h. Abnormal voice sound, clearer transmission of whispered voice sound
9. Whispered pectoriloquy	i. Normal breath sound, with inspiration less than expiration; heard over trachea
10. Bronchophony	j. Normal breath sound with inspiration greater than expiration; heard in most lung fields

4. Mabel Terranova, age 78, is admitted to your unit with a diagnosis of aspiration pneumonia of the right middle lobe. She has a history of cerebrovascular accident and difficulty swallowing. While eating lunch, she began to choke and have respiratory difficulty. Considering Mrs. Terranova's age, what normal differences might you expect to find when assessing her respiratory system?

_____

_____

5. Mrs. Terranova's extremities are pale and dusky. How would you differentiate central cyanosis from peripheral cyanosis?

_____

_____

6. Cyanotic color changes are a late sign of hypoxia. What physical findings would reflect early hypoxia?

_____

_____

7. Considering Mrs. Terranova's diagnosis of right middle lobe pneumonia, what sounds might you expect to hear when you auscultate her lungs?

_____

_____

8. On auscultation, you find that Mrs. Terranova's lungs are clear posteriorly. Considering that she has right middle lobe pneumonia, how do you explain these findings?

_____

_____

9. On admission, Mrs. Terranova's pulse oxygen level is 87% on room air (normal pulse oximetry is 100%). Because her oxygen level is low, what changes might you find in her neurological system, integumentary system, and cardiovascular system?

_____

_____

_____

10. Although your assessment focuses on the respiratory system, all systems are related. What assessment findings (subjective or objective) show the relationship between the respiratory system and other systems?

_____

_____

_____

Name: _____	*Date:* _____
Course: _____	*Instructor:* _____

Abnormal Case Study: Raymond Augustus

Raymond Augustus, a 65-year-old black man, is admitted to the respiratory unit with exacerbation of emphysema. He has had the disease for 10 years and is well known to the staff, having been in and out of the hospital several times. Recently, his hospitalizations have become more frequent. A frail, thin man on oxygen, he is obviously short of breath at rest with pursed-lip breathing. His wife, who accompanies him, comments, "Here we go again!" You take him to his room and make him as comfortable as possible before beginning his admission assessment. Because Mr. Augustus is in mild respiratory distress, you postpone taking a complete history and focus on his chief complaint.

Health History

Chief complaint:

"I can't get my breath and I have a cough."

Symptom analysis:

P—Increased shortness of breath; breathes better when sitting.

Q—Feels like "I can't get enough air."

R—"It's my breathing; my chest is sore from coughing, and I'm so tired."

S—On a scale from 1 to 10, with 10 being the worst, how disabling is this problem? +10

T—Diagnosed with emphysema 10 years ago, has gotten progressively worse to point where he has shortness of breath at rest.

Current health history:

Shortness of breath when performing ADL (grade 3). You compare this with the client's last admission 7 months ago and see that at that time he had shortness of breath with mild activity (grade 2). This helps you determine progression of disease and its effect on the client's life.

- Dyspnea on exertion and orthopnea. Client uses four pillows at night to sleep.
- Productive cough with a large amount of thick, foul-smelling, yellow sputum. Cough sounds congested and had acute onset. *Note:* Mr. Augustus has emphysema; he is not a mucus producer.
- Weight gain of 5 lb in past week; feet are also swollen.
- Before onset of productive cough, client's three grandchildren had visited, and two had colds.
- Client's chest is sore from coughing, and he complains of fatigue.

11. Based on this information, what do you think triggered this current exacerbation?

_____

_____

12. What do you think caused the 5-lb weight gain and swollen feet?

_____

_____

Complete Health History

When the client's condition stabilizes, proceed with a complete health history.

Past health history:

- Multiple admissions over past 10 years for emphysema.
- Received flu shot in October of this year.
- Current medications include a bronchodilator, diuretic, potassium supplement, and "heart pill."

Family history:

- Father had emphysema.

Psychosocial profile:

- *Nutritional patterns:* Poor appetite because eating tires him and he becomes short of breath.
- *Recreation/hobbies:* Loves to fish, but this is becoming more difficult because of illness.
- *Occupational health patterns:* Client was a truck driver forced into early retirement because of emphysema. He experienced possible exposure to air pollutants secondary to job.
- *Environmental health patterns:* Lives in city in a two-story duplex with hot air heat and no central air conditioning. May be exposed to air pollutants secondary to urban residence and home heating system.
- *Roles/relationships:* Lives with wife of 45 years, who is primary support person and caregiver. They rarely socialize with friends and family because of his medical problems and have not been sexually active for some time because of his fatigue and breathing difficulties.

Physical Assessment

- *General appearance:* Appears older than stated age of 65 years; frail; facial expression tired and slightly anxious; position of comfort—tripod.

- *Vital signs:* Temperature 100.2°F; pulse 98 beats/min, regular; respirations 28/min, shallow with effort and prolonged expiratory phase; BP 150/94 mm Hg; weight 115 lb (underweight); height 5 feet, 7 inches.
- *Inspection:*
- *Mental status:* Awake, alert, and oriented × 4 (person, place, time, situation); fatigue.
- *Integumentary:* Skin gray-brown; mucous membranes pale and gray.
- *HEENT:* Trachea midline; positive pursed-lip breathing, neck vein distention, and hypertrophy of neck muscles.
- *Chest:* Anteroposterior:lateral 1:1, barrel chest; costal angle > 90 degrees; symmetrical rise and fall of chest, but decreased excursion at bases; positive use of accessory muscles; skin intact; prominent ribs and intercostals, but no retraction; no spinal deformities.
- *Extremities:* Capillary refill > 6 seconds; positive clubbing; nail beds pale and gray; pedal edema.
- *Palpation:*
- Trachea midline.
- Chest nontender.
- Decreased excursion at bases.
- Increased tactile fremitus over upper lobes.
- *Percussion:*
- Level of diaphragm T12 posterior.
- Hyperresonance at bases; dullness over upper lobes.
- Diaphragmatic excursion: no change between inspiration and expiration.
- *Auscultation:*
- Decreased breath sounds at bases.
- Scattered rhonchi and expiratory wheezes throughout lung fields.

13. What signs/symptoms would you expect to see in a client with nail clubbing?

HYPOXIA, FATIGUE, SHORTNESS OF BREATH, CENTRAL &
PERIPHERAL CYNOSIS.

14. How would you explain the fact that Mr. Augustus's diaphragm is at T12 level with no change in diaphragmatic excursion?

EMPHYSEMA- OVERINFLATION OF LUNGS, PUSHES DIAPHRAM ↓
BECAUSE DIAPHRAM OVERINFLATED, NO CHANGE SEEN

15. What assessment findings are consistent with Mr. Augustus's diagnosis of emphysema?

BARREL CHEST, COSTAL ANGLE ↑ 90°, SHORTNESS OF BREATH,
HYPERRESONCE AT BASES, ↓ BREATH SOUNDS.

16. Cluster the supporting data for the following nursing diagnoses:

a. Ineffective airway clearance related to increased secretions and fatigue.

PRODUCTIVE COUGH, SOB, RESP RATE 28, MUCUS, SHORT
OF BREATH & LUNG SOUNDS

b. Impaired gas exchange related to alveoli destruction.

ON OXYGEN, SOB, IRREGULAR BREATHING, BRONCHIAL DILATER

c. Nutrition less than body requirements related to (dyspnea.) _DIFF. BREATHING._
LOWERED APPETITE, DIFF EATING & BREATHING STIMULTANEOUSLY, SOB
WEIGHT DECREASING.

17. Identify any additional nursing diagnoses for Mr. Augustus.

18. *Word search:* Find the following words in the puzzle: alveoli, asthma, bronchial, egophony, lobe, lung, trachea, vesicular, wheeze.

```
Y  Y  N  O  H  P  O  L  B  Y
L  L  O  B  E  B  W  H  I  Y
W  U  T  R  A  C  H  E  A  N
I  N  E  O  P  W  E  E  R  O
E  G  O  N  P  H  E  E  A  H
U  L  U  C  G  E  Z  Z  C  P
E  V  W  H  E  E  Z  E  H  O
V  E  S  I  C  U  L  A  R  G
U  T  R  A  S  T  H  M  A  E
A  S  A  L  V  E  O  L  I  B
```

Name:	Date:
Course:	Instructor:

Student Lab Sheet: Assessment of the Respiratory System

Health History

Biographical data:

Current health status: symptom analysis (PQRST):

- Cough
- Dyspnea (difficulty breathing, shortness of breath)
- Chest pain
- Related symptoms (edema and fatigue)

Past health history:

- Childhood illnesses
- Hospitalizations
- Surgeries
- Serious injuries/chronic illness
- Immunizations
- Allergies (food, drugs, environmental)
- Medications (prescribed and OTC)
- Recent travel/military service

Family history:

Review of systems:

- General health status
- HEENT
- Cardiovascular
- Gastrointestinal
- Genitourinary
- Musculoskeletal
- Neurological
- Endocrine
- Lymphatic/hematological

Psychosocial profile:

- Health practices and beliefs/self-care activities
- Typical day
- Nutritional patterns (24-hour recall)
- Activity/exercise patterns
- Recreation, pets, hobbies
- Sleep/rest patterns
- Personal habits (tobacco, alcohol, caffeine, and drugs)
- Occupational health patterns
- Socioeconomic status
- Environmental health patterns
- Roles, relationships, self-concept
- Cultural/religious influences
- Family roles/relationships
- Sexuality patterns
- Social supports
- Stress/coping

Physical Assessment

General survey:

- Vital signs
- Height
- Weight

Head-to-toe scan:

- General health status
- Integumentary
- HEENT
- Cardiovascular
- Abdomen
- Genitourinary
- Musculoskeletal
- Neurological

Assessing the Respiratory System

Area/Physical Assessment Skill	Assessment	Normal Findings Developmental/Cultural Variations	Student's Findings
Inspection	**Anterior/posterior/lateral** **Compare side to side, work apex to base** **Position: sitting**	LOOK AT CHEST EXPANSION (LOOKING)	
Chest	Assess respiratory rate, rhythm, depth, symmetry of chest movements	Respiratory rate varies with age. Respirations quiet, symmetrical, with regular rhythm and depth	
	Assess anteroposterior:lateral ratio, costal angle, spinal deformities, muscles for breathing, and condition of skin	Anteroposterior:lateral ratio 1:2, costal angle < 90 degrees, no barrel chest or spinal deformities	
		No retraction or use of accessory muscles, skin intact	
		Senile emphysema, increased	
		Anteroposterior:lateral ratio may be seen in older clients	
		Costal angle increases during pregnancy	
		Women are more thoracic breathers; men and infants are more abdominal breathers	
Palpation	**Anterior/posterior/lateral** **Compare side to side, apex to base**		
Trachea	Place fingers on either side of trachea to assess position	Trachea midline, no deviation	

Chest	Assess for chest tenderness, masses, crepitus Assess excursion at bases if abnormal, assess apices Assess tactile fremitus estimate level of diaphragm, note increased or decreased areas of fremitus **Use balls or ulnar surface of your hands; have client say "99"**		Chest nontender, no masses or crepitus Symmetrical excursion anteriorly and posteriorly. No lags Tactile fremitus equal bilaterally, anteriorly, and posteriorly
Percussion	**Use indirect (mediate) percussion** **Anterior/posterior/lateral** **Compare side to side, apex to base**		
Chest	Note general percussion sound of chest To assess diaphragmatic excursion, percuss level of diaphragm on full expiration and full inspiration, then measure		Anterior chest: resonance to second intercostal space (ICS) on the left, to fourth ICS on right Lateral chest: resonance to eighth ICS Posterior chest: resonance to T12 Diaphragmatic excursion 3–6 cm bilaterally
Auscultation	**Use diaphragm of stethoscope. Have client take slow, deep breaths through mouth** **Anterior/posterior/lateral** **Compare side to side, apex to base**		

Assessing the Respiratory System (Continued)

Area/Physical Assessment Skill	Assessment	Normal Findings Developmental/Cultural Variations	Student's Findings
Breath sounds	**Listen through one full respiratory cycle at each site** Assess normal breath sounds, abnormal sounds, and adventitious sounds (crackles, rhonchi, wheezes, pleural friction rub). Assess for abnormal voice sounds if indicated **Note relationship of inspiration to expiration, pitch, intensity, and location of sounds**	All lungs fields clear to auscultation Bronchial breath sounds heard over trachea Bronchovesicular breath sounds heard over manubrium/sternum anteriorly and between scapula posteriorly Vesicular sounds heard in most lung fields No abnormal or adventitious breath sounds No abnormal voice sounds, egophony, bronchophony, or whispered pectoriloquy	

Pertinent Health History Findings:

Pertinent Physical Assessment Findings:

Nursing Diagnoses (actual or potential) with Clustered Data:

Name: _____	Date: _____
Course: _____	Instructor: _____

Self-Evaluation Exercise

Respiratory System	YES	NO	NEED MORE PRACTICE
1. Applies knowledge of the respiratory system anatomy and physiology in performing a respiratory assessment.			
2. Applies growth and development principles as applicable to the respiratory system.			
3. Considers cultural variations as indicated when performing a respiratory assessment.			
4. Gathers all equipment necessary to perform a respiratory assessment.			
5. Obtains history specific to assessment of the respiratory system.			
6. Performs a physical assessment of the respiratory system, including: • General survey and head-to-toe scan • Inspection • Palpation • Percussion • Auscultation			
7. Documents respiratory assessment findings.			
8. Identifies normal/abnormal findings.			
9. Clusters pertinent subjective/objective data.			
10. Identifies actual/potential health problems and states them as nursing diagnoses with supporting data.			

Chapter 12

Assessing the Cardiovascular System

Name: _____	Date: _____
Course: _____	Instructor: _____

1. Anatomy review: Label the following structures.

- Right atrium
- Right ventricle
- Right pulmonary arteries
- Right pulmonary veins
- Mitral (AV) valve
- Aortic arch
- Aortic semilunar valve
- Pulmonary semilunar valve
- Thoracic aorta
- Inferior vena cava
- Interventricular septum
- Myocardium
- Epicardium
- Tricuspid (AV) valve
- Superior vena cava
- Subepicardial fat and connective tissue
- Fibrous pericardium
- Coronary artery and vein
- Epicardium or visceral pericardium
- Serous pericardium parietal layer

- Left atrium
- Left ventricle
- Left pulmoanry arteries
- Left pulmonary veins
- Pericardium
- Pericardial space
- Endocardium

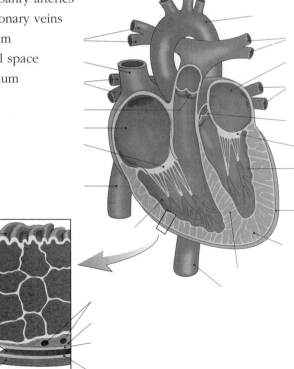

- Atrioventricular node

- Superior vena cava

- Sinoatrial node

- Purkinje fibers

- Left atrium

- Right atrium

- Atrioventricular bundle (bundle of His)

- Right ventricle

- Left ventricle

- Myocardium

- Left bundle branch

- Right bundle branch

- Bachmann's bundle

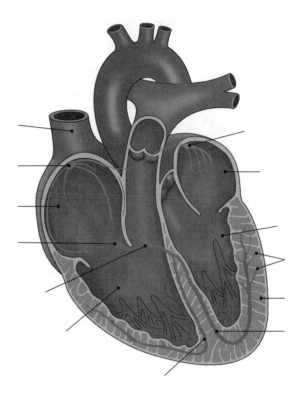

- Left base

- Apex

- Left lateral sternal border

- Erb's point

- Right base

- Aortic valve

- Mitral valve

- Tricuspid valve

- Xiphoid

- Pulmonic valve

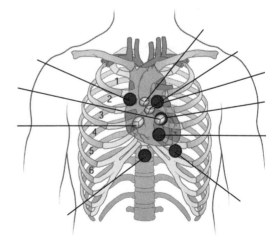

2. Match the structure in the first column to its description in the second column.

Structure	Description
1. Myocardium	a. Valve between right atrium and right ventricle
2. Endocardium	b. Pacemaker of heart at rate of 60–100 beats/min
3. Pericardial space	c. Pumps blood to the systemic circulation
4. Right atrium	d. Paces heart at 40–60 beats/min
5. Left atrium	e. Space between parietal and visceral layer
6. Sinoatrial node	f. Muscle layer of heart
7. Right ventricle	g. Smooth inner layer of heart
8. Left ventricle	h. Pumps blood to pulmonary circulation
9. Tricuspid valve	i. Major vein of head
10. Jugular	j. Major artery that provides blood supply to head
11. Aortic valve	k. Valve between right ventricle and pulmonary artery
12. Mitral valve	l. Valve between left ventricle and aorta
13. Carotid artery	m. Receives oxygenated blood from pulmonary veins
14. Pulmonic valve	n. Valve between left atrium and left ventricle
15. Atrioventricular node	o. Receives blood from superior and inferior vena cavae

3. Match the heart sound in the first column to its description in the second column.

Heart Sounds	Description
1. S_1	a. S_1, S_2, S_3, S_4
2. S_2	b. High-pitched systolic sound occurring when aortic or pulmonic valves open; associated with mitral valve prolapse
3. S_3	c. High-pitched sound occurring when mitral and tricuspid valves close
4. S_4	d. Sound created by turbulent flow
5. Ejection click	e. Each component of S_1 is heard
6. Opening snap	f. Each component of S_2 is heard
7. Split S_1	g. High-pitched sound occurring when aortic and pulmonic valves close
8. Split S_2	h. Low-pitched early diastolic sound that is sign of "distressed" heart; heard with congestive heart failure
9. Murmur	i. Low-pitched late diastolic sound that is sign of "stressed" heart; often heard with HTN
10. Quadruple rhythm	j. High-pitched diastolic sound occurring when mitral or tricuspid valves open

4. When auscultating at the apex, which heart sound is normally louder, S_1 or S_2? Which sound is louder when auscultating at the base?

_____

_____

5. You know that S_1 and S_2 can split. At what site would you expect to hear a normal split S_1? A split S_2?

_____

_____

6. A split S_2 is often easier to detect than a split S_1 because of a respiratory variation. What effects do respirations have on S_2?

_____

_____

7. Robert Simons, age 55, presents in the ED with a chief complaint of chest pain. On admission, his vital signs are BP 170/118 mm Hg; pulse 123 beats/min, regular; respirations 24/min. His skin is gray, diaphoretic, and cool. The cardiac monitor shows sinus tachycardia with elevated ST waves. Mr. Simons is started on a nitroglycerin drip. With tachycardia, it is difficult to differentiate S_1 from S_2. Name three ways to establish the timing of the cardiac cycle to differentiate the heart sounds.

_____

_____

8. Mr. Simons also has a history of HTN. Considering his history of HTN and his possible myocardial infarction, what additional heart sound might you expect to hear and why?

_____

_____

9. Mr. Simons develops congestive heart failure. What additional heart sound might you hear and why?

_____

_____

10. You assess Mr. Simons's jugular venous pressure. There are four ways to differentiate the venous pulsation from the carotid pulsation. What are they?

_____

_____

11. What two points are used to measure jugular venous pressure?

_____

_____

12. Establishing timing in the cardiac cycle is essential in identifying heart sounds. Describe how you would differentiate the following sounds. Include the timing of the sound in the cardiac cycle, whether the sound is systolic or diastolic, the area where the sound is heard best, and the pitch of the sound (high or low).

    a. A split S_1 from an S_4.

    _____

    b. A split S_1 from an ejection click.

    _____

    c. A split S_2 from an S_3.

    _____

    d. A split S_3 from an opening snap.

    _____

13. Mr. Simons is admitted to the cardiac care unit until his condition stabilizes. On his third postinfarction day, he develops pericarditis. What additional heart sound would you expect to hear? Describe the sound, and identify the site where you would expect to hear it.

    _____

    _____

14. Karen Kelly is a 35-year-old woman with a history of mitral valve prolapse. On examination, you detect a murmur. Name five causes of murmurs.

    _____

    _____

15. List five characteristics used to describe a murmur.

    _____

    _____

16. A murmur may be innocent or indicate pathology. Name two characteristics of murmurs that indicate pathology.

    _____

    _____

17. Part of the vascular examination includes auscultation for carotid bruits. When auscultating, what instructions should you give the patient? What part of the stethoscope is best for detecting bruits?

    _____

    _____

18. Although your assessment focuses on the cardiovascular system, all systems are related. What assessment findings (subjective or objective) show the relationship between the cardiovascular system and other systems?

    _____

    _____

    _____

Name: _____ Date: _____

Course: _____ Instructor: _____

Abnormal Case Study: Henry Brusca

Henry Brusca, a 72-year-old white man, presents in the ED complaining of chest discomfort. He says it started 2 hours ago, after he finished dinner and then awakened from a nap. Mr. Brusca is well known to you. He has been treated for HTN for the past 4 years. In the ED, he is given aspirin and started on a nitroglycerin drip. An ECG and serum cardiac enzyme test are obtained. Mr. Brusca is admitted to the cardiac care unit with the diagnosis of anterior wall myocardial infarction. He asks you, "Am I going to die?" His condition is critical, so you obtain a focused history.

Health History

Chief complaint:

"I have terrible chest pain."

Symptom analysis:

P—Discomfort started after eating dinner; pain woke him up from a nap; had large meal. States, "I thought it was indigestion, so took some antacids, but nothing seemed to make it better."

Q—"Feels like someone sitting on my chest—pressure!"

R—"Right here in the middle on my chest." No radiation; shortness of breath at rest.

S—10/10.

T—"It started about 0.5 hour after dinner. I never had indigestion this bad before."

Complete Health History

When the patient's condition stabilizes, proceed with the complete health history.

Biographical data:

- A 72-year-old white man, married, father of seven grown children.
- Self-employed entrepreneur; BS degree in engineering.
- Born and raised in the United States, Italian descent, Catholic religion.

- Blue Cross/Blue Shield medical insurance plan.
- Referral: follow-up by primary care physician.
- Source: self, reliable.

Past health history:

- Previous ECG revealed left ventricular hypertrophy.
- Hospitalized for HTN.
- No known food, drug, or environmental allergies.
- No other previous medical problem.
- No prescribed medications except enalapril (Vasotec), 5 mg twice a day (took today's dose), and weekly use of antacid for indigestion.

Family history:

- Positive family history of HTN, myocardial infarction, and cerebrovascular accident.

Physical Assessment

- *General appearance:* Well-developed, well-groomed 72-year-old white man, in obvious discomfort. Sitting upright clutching chest. Alert and responsive, oriented × 4, affect anxious.
- *Vital signs:* Temperature 100°F; pulse 115 beats/min, strong with occasional extra beat; respirations 28/min, shallow; BP 170/105 mm Hg; height 6 feet; weight 275 lb.

- *Integumentary:* Skin intact, pale/ashen, diaphoretic, good turgor; mucous membranes pale gray and moist; poor capillary refill, negative clubbing; skin cool, pale, shiny, and hairless on lower extremities.

- *HEENT:* Eyes: Negative periorbital edema; positive arcus senilis; funduscopic, positive atrioventricular knicking and cotton wool; negative papilledema and hemorrhages. Thyroid not palpable.

- *Respiratory:* Lungs: bibasilar crackles, decreased breath sounds at bases because of guarded respirations; anteroposterior:lateral ratio 1:2.

- *Peripheral-vascular:* +1 peripheral pulses.

- *Gastrointestinal:* Abdomen large, round, soft, nontender; positive bowel sounds; negative hepatomegaly; positive pulsation in epigastric area; negative bruits or thrills.

- *Musculoskeletal/neurological:* Sensory intact, +2 deep tendon reflexes (DTRs), muscle strength equal, positive hand grip, lower extremities +4/5 muscle strength.

Focused Physical Assessment Findings

Neck vessels:

- Positive carotid pulsation, +2; symmetrical with smooth, sharp upstroke and rapid descent; artery stiff; negative for thrills and bruits.

- Neck vein distention, jugular venous pressure at 30 degrees > 3 cm, positive abdominal jugular reflux.

Precordium:

- Positive sustained pulsations displaced lateral to apex, point of maximum impulse (PMI) 3 cm with increased amplitude.

- Slight pulsations also appreciated at left lateral sternal border (LLSB) and base, but not as pronounced.

- Negative thrills; cardiac borders percussed third, fourth, and fifth ICS to the left of the midclavicular line.

- Heart sounds appreciated with tachycardia and irregular rhythm at apex $S_1 > S_2$ and $S_1 < S_2$ at base; positive S_3 and S_4.

- S_2 negative split, at base left $S_1 < S_2$ negative split, at base right $S_1 < S_2$ with an accentuated S_2; negative for murmurs and rubs.

19. What areas are of major concern and warrant continued assessment?

    CARDIOVASCULAR, RESPITORY

20. The PMI is enlarged. What factors may account for this finding?

    HTN, ↓ LEFT VENTRICULAR HYPERTROPHY

21. Mr. Brusca's physical findings also reveal neck vein distention and an elevated jugular venous pressure. How would you explain these findings?

    SIGNS OF RIGHT-SIDED HEART FAILURE

22. How would you explain the presence of an S_3 and S_4 on physical examination?

    S4 COULD BE ASSOCIATED WITH HTN OR ACUTE MYOCARDIAL INFARCTION & S3 COULD BE ASSOCIATED WITH CONGESTIVE HEART FAILURE.

23. Cluster the data for the following nursing diagnoses:

a. Pain related to tissue ischemia.

CHEST DISCOMFORT, ANXIOUS, CLUTCHING CHEST, ↑ BP, PULSE
RESP.

b. Anxiety related to threat of dying.

ANXIOUS, "AM I GOING TO DIE" ↑ VITALS

c. Ineffective tissue perfusion related to decreased blood flow.

SKIN PALE, ASHEN, MUCOUS MEMBRANES PALE GRAY
SKIN COOL, HAIRLESS ON LOWER EXTREM.

d. Decreased cardiac output related to altered myocardial contractility.

TACHYCARDIA, IRREGULAR RHYTHM, HTN, ECG SHOWS MYOCARDIAL
INFARC.

24. Which of the above-listed diagnoses would be of highest priority? Why?

DECREASED CARDIAC OUTPUT & INEFFECTIVE TISSUE PERFUSION.
IMPROVING CARDIAC OUTPUT & TISSUE PERFUSION

25. Identify any additional nursing diagnoses for Mr. Brusca.

26. *Word search:* Find the following words in the puzzle: aorta, artery, bruit, carotid, heart, heave, mitral, murmur, vein, ventricle.

M	C	A	M	T	Y	L	A	H	E
U	A	R	I	C	L	H	Y	L	A
M	I	T	R	A	L	E	C	M	T
U	B	E	T	R	I	I	B	U	R
R	U	R	A	O	R	T	A	R	I
B	H	Y	U	T	H	H	I	M	V
V	E	O	N	I	T	E	R	U	M
H	A	E	T	D	T	A	T	R	I
A	V	E	I	N	R	R	A	M	E
L	E	Y	P	I	A	T	I	E	V

Name: _____ Date: _____

Course: _____ Instructor: _____

Student Lab Sheet: Assessment of the Cardiovascular System

Health History

Biographical data:

Current health status: symptom analysis (PQRST):

- Chest pain
- Dyspnea
- Cough
- Edema
- Syncope
- Palpitations
- Fatigue
- Extremity changes

Past health history:

- Childhood illnesses
- Hospitalizations
- Surgeries
- Serious injuries/chronic illness
- Immunizations
- Allergies (food, drugs, environmental)
- Medications
- Recent travel/military service

Family history:

Review of systems:

- General health status
- HEENT
- Respiratory
- Gastrointestinal
- Genitourinary
- Musculoskeletal
- Neurological
- Endocrine
- Lymphatic/hematological

Psychosocial profile:

- Health practices and beliefs/self-care activities
- Typical day
- Nutritional patterns (24-hour recall)
- Activity/exercise patterns
- Recreation, pets, hobbies
- Sleep/rest patterns
- Personal habits (tobacco, alcohol, caffeine, and drugs)
- Occupational health patterns
- Socioeconomic status
- Environmental health patterns
- Roles, relationships, self-concept
- Cultural/religious influences
- Family roles/relationships
- Sexuality patterns
- Social supports
- Stress/coping

Physical Assessment

General survey:

- Vital signs
- Height
- Weight

Head-to-toe scan:

- Integumentary
- HEENT
- Respiratory
- Abdomen
- Genitourinary
- Musculoskeletal
- Neurological

Assessment of the Cardiovascular System

Area/Physical Assessment Skill	Assessment	Normal Findings Developmental/Cultural Variations	Student's Findings
Inspection	**Positions: sitting, supine, left lateral recumbent**		
Neck vessels: carotid arteries and jugular veins	Differentiate carotid pulsations from venous pulsations	Visible carotid pulsation. No neck vein distention. Jugular venous pressure at 45 degree angle < 3 cm	
	Jugular pulsations easily obliterated, affected by position, respirations, undulating wave	Carotid pulsation with one positive wave	
	Measure jugular venous pressure with client at a 45 degree angle at sternal angle (angle of Louis)	Jugular pulsation undulated	
Precordium	Note pulsations in apex, left lateral sternal border, bases, and xyphoid or epigastric areas	Positive pulsation noted at apex	
		Slight pulsation noted at bases in thin adults and children	
Palpation	**Palpate each carotid separately**	Slight epigastric pulsations may be noted	
Neck vessels: carotid arteries and jugular veins	Note rate, rhythm, amplitude, contour, symmetry, elasticity, thrills	Carotids: Rate age dependent; regular rhythm, +2 amplitude, +3 high-output states, equal contour, smooth upstroke with less acute descent; large pulse wave may be seen in elderly and during exercise	
	If you feel a carotid thrill, listen for a bruit	Carotids soft and pliable; may be stiff and cordlike in elderly. No thrills	
	Palpate jugular veins and check direction of fill. Check for abdominojugular (hepatojugular) reflux	Jugulars easily obliterated and fill appropriately. Negative abdominojugular reflux	

Technique	Normal Findings
Precordium Palpate apex, left lateral sternal border, bases, and xyphoid or epigastric areas Note size, duration, and diffusion of impulses Note thrills, lifts, or heaves **If you palpate a thrill, listen for a murmur**	PMI at apex 1–2 cm, nonsustained, or may normally be nonpalpable Slight epigastric pulsation, no diffusion No pulsations noted at base and LLSB Small nonsustained impulses may be palpable at base and LLSB of thin adults and children PMI may be displaced laterally and to left during last trimester of pregnancy Increased amplitude in high-output states No lifts, heaves, or thrills
Percussion **Use indirect (mediate) percussion**	
Precordium Percuss from anterior axillary line to sternum at fifth ICS	Dullness noted third, fourth, and fifth ICS to left of sternum at midclavicular line
Auscultation **Listen with bell (light pressure) and diaphragm (heavy pressure) of stethoscope at all sites**	
Carotids Listen for bruits with bell of stethoscope **Have client hold breath when auscultating for carotid bruits**	Negative carotid bruits Carotid bruit may be normal in children and with high-output states

Assessment of the Cardiovascular System (*Continued*)

Area/Physical Assessment Skill	Assessment	Normal Findings Developmental/Cultural Variations	Student's Findings
Jugular veins	Have client hold breath when auscultating with bell for venous hums **To differentiate venous hum from transmitted murmur, remember that venous hum disappears when pressure is applied to jugular vein**	Negative venous hum Venous hum may be normal finding in children	
Precordium Apex: fifth ICS, left midclavicular line LLSB: fourth to fifth ICS, lateral sternal border Erb's point: third ICS, lateral sternal border Base left: second ICS, lateral sternal border Base right: second ICS, right sternal border Xyphoid area	**Auscultate in sitting, supine, and left lateral recumbent positions** Listen to S_1, S_2, splits, and extra sounds (S_3, S_4, OS ejection click, murmurs, pericardial rubs) Note rate, rhythm, pitch, intensity, duration, timing in cardiac cycle, quality, location, and radiation **Abnormal aortic murmurs heard best at Erb's point** Grade murmurs on 1–6 scale. *A diastolic murmur or murmur > grade 3/6 is never innocent*	Apex: Rate/age dependent, rhythm regular, high-pitched, systolic, short duration, 3/6 intensity, $S_1 > S_2$, accentuated S_1 in high-output states LLSB: $S_1 >$ or $= S_2$, split S_1 possible Base left: $S_1 < S_2$, split S_2 during inspiration Base right: $S_1 < S_2$ No extra sounds	

Pertinent Health History Findings:

Pertinent Physical Assessment Findings:

Nursing Diagnoses (actual or potential) with Clustered Data:

Name: _____   *Date:* _____

Course: _____   *Instructor:* _____

Self-Evaluation Exercise

Cardiovascular System	YES	NO	NEED MORE PRACTICE
1. Applies knowledge of the cardiovascular system anatomy and physiology in performing a cardiovascular assessment			
2. Applies growth and development principles as applicable to the cardiovascular system.			
3. Considers cultural variations as indicated when performing a cardiovascular assessment			
4. Gathers all equipment necessary to perform a cardiovascular assessment			
5. Obtains history specific to assessment of the cardiovascular system			
6. Performs a physical assessment of the cardiovascular system, including: • General survey and head-to-toe scan • Inspection • Palpation • Percussion • Auscultation			
7. Documents cardiovascular assessment findings			
8. Identifies normal/abnormal findings.			
9. Clusters pertinent subjective/objective data.			
10. Identifies actual/potential health problems and states them as nursing diagnoses with supporting data.			

Chapter 13

Assessing the Peripheral-Vascular and Lymphatic Systems

Name: _____	Date: _____
Course: _____	Instructor: _____

1. Anatomy review: Label the following pulse sites

   - Temporal
   - Carotid
   - Brachial
   - Radial
   - Ulnar
   - Popliteal
   - Dorsalis pedis
   - Posterior tibial
   - Femoral

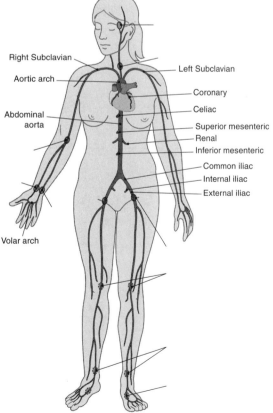

Right Subclavian

Aortic arch

Abdominal aorta

Volar arch

Left Subclavian

Coronary

Celiac

Superior mesenteric

Renal

Inferior mesenteric

Common iliac

Internal iliac

External iliac

2. Match the structure in the first column to its specific function in the second column.

Structure	Function
1. Carotid artery	a. Lymphatic tissue found in oropharynx
2. Peyer's patch	b. Drain arms
3. Jugular veins	c. Provides blood supply to brain
4. Thymus	d. Organ in left upper quadrant of abdomen that produces lymphocytes and monocytes
5. Spleen	e. Drain head
6. Subclavian veins	f. Cluster of lymphatic tissue in intestines
7. Femoral artery	g. Drain legs
8. Brachial artery	h. Provides blood supply to legs
9. Tonsils	i. Provides blood supply to arms
10. Iliac veins	j. Lymphatic tissue in thorax that helps with T-cell differentiation

3. You are working in an HTN clinic. Describe the technique you should use to avoid the auscultatory gap when measuring BP.

_____

_____

4. What three positions should the client be in when you measure for orthostatic drops in BP?

_____

5. If your client has a true orthostatic drop, what changes would you expect to find?

_____

_____

6. You are doing a vascular assessment on Joe McCloskey, a 70-year-old man with a history of diabetes mellitus and peripheral-vascular disease. Identify five characteristics you should include in the pulse assessment.

_____

_____

7. Considering Mr. McCloskey's age, what would you expect to be a normal variation of the pulse assessment associated with aging?

_____

8. Mr. McCloskey tells you that he has an ulcer on his foot caused by vascular problems and diabetes. How do the signs of arterial insufficiency differ from those of venous insufficiency?

_____

_____

9. What additional test could you do to assess the circulation in Mr. McCloskey's feet?

_____

10. Patty Hoffman, age 14, has mononucleosis and associated lymphadenopathy. Name five characteristics that you should note when describing palpable lymph nodes.

_____

_____

11. What would you expect to find when assessing Patty's lymph nodes?

_____

_____

12. Lymph nodes normally vary depending on the person's age. What variations would you expect to see in a young child? In an older adult?

_____

_____

13. Although your assessment focuses on the peripheral-vascular and lymphatic systems, all systems are related. What assessment findings (subjective or objective) show the relationship between the peripheral-vascular and lymphatic systems and other systems?

_____

_____

_____

Name: _____	*Date:* _____
Course: _____	*Instructor:* _____

Abnormal Case Study: Morris Hart

Morris Hart, a 58-year-old, married black man, is admitted to your medical unit. He has a history of coronary artery disease, HTN, and diabetes. Mr. Hart describes himself as being "in fairly good health" and mentions that he has worked hard to develop a healthy lifestyle. He hasn't had anymore "chest pain attacks" and he has been monitoring his BP and his blood sugar at home. He is admitted because of intermittent claudication and pain in his left leg and small open ulcers on two of his toes.

    Helpful Hint: Claudication alone is thought to be benign in regard to limb loss, and with lifestyle modification, symptoms remain the same or improve in 80% of clients.

Health History

Chief complaint:

"My left leg hurts, and I have two sores on my toes that won't heal."

Symptom analysis:

P—Client states that pain occurs sooner when he is walking on an incline or climbing stairs. Reports that pain disappears when he stops walking. He hasn't taken any medications to relieve the pain.

Q—Client describes pain as a "tightening pressure" and says he sometimes has a sharp, "cramplike" sensation. Says that several months ago pain occurred only occasionally, but now it occurs almost daily and after walking much shorter distances. It is affecting his ability to do his job.

R—Says that pain is in muscles of calves, thighs, and buttocks on both sides, but left side is worse than right. Besides leg pain, client has noticed a small ulcer on great toe of his left foot.

T—Has had increasing difficulty walking over past 6 months. Pain usually starts after he has walked about 50 yards and lasts 10 minutes after he stops walking.

Current health status:

- *Intermittent claudication:* Progressive worsening over last 6 months that is more painful in left leg.

- *HTN:* Client is on an angiotensin-converting enzyme inhibitor medication to control BP. He takes his BP two to three times weekly using a home monitor kit. His usual reading is about 150 to 160/90 mm Hg.

- *Diabetes mellitus:* Client has been a diabetic for 10 years. He takes an oral hyperglycemic agent twice daily and monitors his diet to keep blood glucose under control. Reports a usual fasting blood glucose (before breakfast) between 150 and 160 mg/dL.

- *Coronary artery disease:* Client had a few episodes of chest pain several years ago and was diagnosed with stable angina. Has sublingual nitroglycerin to take if pain occurs and takes one aspirin daily. Hasn't needed nitroglycerin for more than 1 year.

- *Smoking:* Smoked two packs of cigarettes a day for 30 years. After chest pain episodes, he tried several times to stop smoking but has only been able to cut down to one pack a day.

Family history:

- Father died of an acute myocardial infarction at age 57.

Mother is alive but had a cerebrovascular accident at age 62 and has been a type 2 diabetic for 15 years.

Psychosocial profile:

- *Nutritional patterns:* Tries hard to follow diet dietitian gave him when he was first diagnosed with diabetes. Says it has been hard to "eat healthy" lately and admits to cheating on his diet lately. Attributes his current high blood glucose values to this situation. Mrs. Hart has been nagging him to watch his diet.

- *Recreation/hobbies:* Is too busy to have any hobbies. After work, he eats dinner and watches television.

- *Occupational health patterns:* Mr. Hart is a salesman for a drug company, which requires long hours and frequent out-of-town travel.

- *Environmental health patterns:* Lives in a ranch-style house in suburbs. Has central heating and air conditioning.

- *Roles/relationships:* Lives with his wife. They have two sons in college who come home summers and holidays. The Harts enjoy going to the movies and out to dinner with friends. They used to take long walks in nice weather, but Mr. Hart's current leg problems have interfered with this activity.

14. From Mr. Hart's history, identify risk factors for vascular disease.

_____

_____

Physical Assessment

- *General appearance:* Well nourished, in no acute distress, slightly anxious.

- *Vital signs:* Afrebrile; pulse 98 beats/min, regular; respirations 16/min, unlabored, BP 150/96 mm Hg; weight 200 lb (overweight); height 5 feet, 9 inches; BMI 29.

- *Inspection:*

- *Head and neck:* No jugular vein distention.

- *Upper extremities:* Skin color uniform; capillary refill < 3 seconds; no edema or skin lesions.

- *Abdomen:* No visible pulsations.

- *Lower extremities:*

- Feet pale on elevation and dusky red on dependency, worse in left leg.

- Skin thin and shiny.

- Patchy hair loss.

- No varicosities.

- No edema.

- Nails thickened.

- Ulcer on lateral side of great toe measuring 2 cm × 2 cm.

Palpation:

- *Head and neck:* Temporal and carotid arteries + 2 bilaterally.

- *Upper extremities:* Brachial, radial, and ulnar pulses easily palpable (+ 2); no abnormal filling on Allen's test.

- *Abdomen:* No abdominal pulsatile mass noted.

- *Lower extremities:*

- Femoral and popliteal pulses easily palpable (+ 2) bilaterally.

- Dorsalis pedis and posterior tibial pulses absent.

- Feet and legs cool, especially on left side.

- Calf circumference: left leg = 20 cm; right leg = 20.5 cm.

Auscultation:

- *Head and neck:* No carotid bruits.

- *Upper extremities:* BP 156/96 mm Hg right arm; 158/94 mm Hg left arm.

- *Abdomen:* No vascular sounds auscultated.

15. What findings suggest arterial insufficiency?

   LEASIONS ON TOES, ABSENT PULSES, THIN, SHINEY SKIN, PATCHY HAIR LOSS,
   THICK NAILS, COLOR CHANGES IN LEGS, COOL FEET.

16. What additional assessment test would help evaluate the circulation in Mr. Hart's lower extremities?

   ANKLE BRACHIAL INDEX.

17. Before treating the lesions on Mr. Hart's toes, it is essential to assess blood flow in the lower extremities. Why?

   BLOOD FLOW MUST BE ADEQUATE TO THE LOWER EXTREMITIES TO
   ENSURE HEALING.

18. Cluster the supporting data for the following nursing diagnoses:

   a. Pain related to ischemia.
      INTERMITTENT CLAUDICATION & CRAMPING NLEGS WHEN WALKING

   b. Altered tissue perfusion related to decreased arterial blood flow.
      INTERMITTENT CLAUDICATION, COOL FEET, ABSENT PEDAL PULSE, THIN, HAIR LOSS

   c. Impaired skin integrity related to decreased peripheral perfusion.
      ULCERS ON TOES

19. Identify any additional nursing diagnoses for Mr. Hart.

   _____

   _____

20. What health promotion topics should you teach Mr. Hart?

   _____

21. Describe a walking program for Mr. Hart and its role.

   _____

   _____

22. Teaching about leg and foot care is an important intervention for clients with peripheral arterial occlusive disease. List key elements of a teaching plan for Mr. Hart.

   _____

   _____

23. *Word jumble:* Unscramble the following words. Then unscramble the circled letters to complete the sentence: Arteries are auscultated for

_____

1. A H I C A Ⓑ L R

2. F O K K O R O F Ⓣ

3. G E R B E Ⓡ U   E D S I S A E

4. Y A N R D Ⓤ A S   S E D I Ⓢ A E

5. N A M S O H   G N S Ⓘ

6. L E L N A   E S T T

7. O P I L E T P L A

8. R F O L A M E

9. I N E V

10. T E R A Y R

Name: _____   Date: _____

Course: _____   Instructor: _____

Student Lab Sheet: Assessment of the Peripheral-Vascular and Lymphatic Systems

Health History

Biographical data:

Current health status: symptom analysis (PQRST):

- Swelling
- Limb pain
- Changes in sensations
- Fatigue

Past health history:

- Childhood illnesses
- Hospitalizations
- Surgeries
- Serious injuries/chronic illness
- Immunizations
- Allergies (food, drugs, environmental)
- Medications (prescribed and OTC)
- Recent travel/military service

Family history:

Review of systems:

- General health status
- HEENT
- Integumentary
- Respiratory
- Cardiovascular
- Gastrointestinal
- Genitourinary
- Musculoskeletal
- Neurological
- Endocrine
- Lymphatic/hematological

Psychosocial profile:

- Health practices and beliefs/self-care activities
- Typical day
- Nutritional patterns (24-hour recall)
- Activity/exercise patterns
- Recreation, pets, hobbies
- Sleep/rest patterns
- Personal habits (tobacco, alcohol, caffeine, and drugs)
- Occupational health patterns
- Socioeconomic status
- Environmental health patterns
- Roles, relationships, self-concept
- Cultural/religious influences
- Family roles/relationships
- Sexuality patterns
- Social supports
- Stress/coping

Physical Assessment

General survey:

- Vital signs
- Height
- Weight

Head-to-toe scan:

- General health status
- Integumentary
- HEENT
- Respiratory
- Abdomen
- Genitourinary
- Neurological

Assessing of the Peripheral-Vascular and Lymphatic Systems

Area/Physical Assessment Skill	Assessment	Normal Findings Developmental/Cultural Variations	Student's Findings
Inspection	**Position: supine and sitting**		
Upper extremities	Note color, edema, erythema, red streaks, lesions, and capillary refill	Skin color uniform; no erythema, red streaks, edema, or lesions	UPPER LIMBS ARE LIGHT TAN IN COLOR, HAIR GROWTH MINIMAL NO REMARKABLE SCARS, ERYTHEMA OR LESIONS.
	Look for edema on most dependent parts of body		CAPILLARY REFILL IMMEDIATE
	If edema present, weigh client daily. Grade edema grade +1 to +4		TEMP OF LIMBS NORMAL
Abdomen	Note shape, arterial pulsation, increased venous pattern, ascites	Abdomen flat or slightly rounded. No increased venous pattern or ascites	SLIGHTLY ROUNDED & MINIMAL VENOUS INCREASE ON BACK OF LEGS.
	If ascites present, do fluid wave test or test for shifting dullness	Slight arterial pulsation noted in epigastric region at midline	
	If large, diffuse arterial pulsation present, do not palpate abdomen		
Lower extremities	Note color, skin condition, hair distribution, varicosities, edema, erythema, red streaks, and lesions	Leg hair evenly distributed; color uniform; no edema, varicosities, erythema, red streaks, or lesions	LIGHT PEDAL PALE, NO SKIN VARIATION; NO EDEMA, HAIR DISTRIBUTION MINIMAL.
	If edema present, measure calf circumference		
	If varicosities present, check venous valve competence with Trendelenburg test or manual compression test		

Palpation	Use light palpation with finger pads	
Pulses: Carotid	Note rate, rhythm, equality, amplitude, elasticity, and thrills	Pulses rate/age dependent, regular, equal, +2, arteries soft and pliable. No thrills
Temporal	Grade amplitude:	Negative Homan's sign
Brachial	0 = absent	**Document pulse amplitudes on a stick figure**
Radial	1 = weak	
Ulnar	2 = normal	
Femoral	3 = full	
Popliteal	4 = bounding	
Dorsalis pedis	**If thrill is present, listen for a bruit**	
Posterior	If indicated, do Allen test to assess arterial flow to hands. If indicated, do color change test or measure ankle-brachial index to assess arterial flow to legs	
Tibialis	If thrombus or thrombophlebitis suspected, test Homan's sign	
Extremities	Assess capillary refill and skin temperature	Positive capillary refill < 3 seconds. Extremities warm bilaterally

Handwritten annotations:

2 – (CAROTID)
      – BRACHIAL
DORSAL PEDAL   LIGHT.

1 – TEMPORAL

CAP REFILL IMMEDIATE

Assessing of the Peripheral-Vascular and Lymphatic System (*Continued*)

Area/Physical Assessment Skill	Assessment	Normal Findings Developmental/Cultural Variations	Student's Findings
Lymph nodes: Cervical Axillary Epitrochlear Inguinal (horizontal and vertical) Popliteal	Note size, shape, symmetry, tenderness, mobility, consistency, delineation, location, erythema, warmth, or increased vascularity	Lymph nodes not palpable. If node is palpable, normal characteristics include: < 1 cm; firm; nontender; round or oval; borders well defined; mobile; no erythema, warmth, or increased vascularity	
Auscultation	**Use bell of stethoscope**		
Arteries	Auscultate for bruits	No bruits	
	Have client hold breath when auscultating for bruits over neck		
BP	Measure BP in both arms, supine, sitting, and, standing	Normal BP age dependent	
	Avoid auscultatory gap by palpating brachial pulse and inflating cuff until pulse is obliterated, then reinflate cuff 30 mm Hg above the point where pulse was obliterated	Adult: systolic < 140 mm Hg, diastolic <90 mm Hg	
		Pulse pressure is one third of systolic pressure	
	Note orthostatic drop of BP **(decrease of systolic by 10–15 mm Hg with increase in pulse rate)**	No orthostatic drop	
		If BP heard down to "0," retake BP and listen for Korotkoff sounds 1, 4 (first diastolic), and 5, then record all three	
	Note pulse pressure **(difference between systolic and diastolic)**		

Pertinent Health History Findings:

_____

Pertinent Physical Assessment Findings:

_____

Nursing Diagnoses (actual or potential) with Clustered Data:

_____

Name: _____   Date: _____

Course: _____   Instructor: _____

Self-Evaluation Exercise

Peripheral-Vascular and Lymphatic Systems	YES	NO	NEED MORE PRACTICE
1. Applies knowledge of peripheral-vascular and lymphatic systems anatomy and physiology in performing an assessment of the peripheral-vascular and lymphatic systems			
2. Applies growth and development principles as applicable to the peripheral-vascular and lymphatic systems			
3. Considers cultural variations as indicated when performing a peripheral-vascular and lymphatic assessment			
4. Gathers all equipment necessary to perform a peripheral-vascular and lymphatic systems assessment			
5. Obtains history specific to assessment of the peripheral-vascular and lymphatic systems			
6. Performs a physical assessment of the peripheral-vascular and lymphatic systems, including: General survey and head-to-toe scan Inspection Palpation Auscultation			
7. Documents peripheral-vascular and lymphatic system assessment findings			
8. Identifies normal/abnormal findings			
9. Clusters pertinent subjective/objective data			
10. Identifies actual/potential health problems and states them as nursing diagnoses with supporting data			

Name: _____	Date: _____
Course: _____	Instructor: _____

Abnormal Case Study: Mary Jane Marshall

Mary Jane Marshall, 45 years old, is scheduled for a lumpectomy of a possibly malignant breast mass. She is married, has two children ages 14 and 12, and works as a freelance commercial artist. She is accompanied by her husband, who seems supportive and concerned. Mrs. Marshall discovered the breast mass during a BSE 2 weeks ago. She is anxious and on the verge of tears, stating, "I'm so afraid it might be cancer."

Health History

Current health status:

Breast mass discovered during BSE.

Past health history:

- No history of breast disease or uterine, ovarian, or colon cancer.
- Menarche age 11.
- Para 2, gravida 2.

Family history:

- Mother and aunt had breast cancer.

Physical Assessment

- Breast mass 4 cm, nontender, irregular, hard, and immobile.
- Anxious, nervous, and tearful.

10. What factors put Mrs. Marshall at risk for breast cancer?

_____

_____

11. Considering Mrs. Marshall's findings, what additional area should you assess?

_____

12. Cluster the supporting data for the following nursing diagnoses:

a. Risk for pain related to surgical incision.

_____

b. Fear related to possible diagnosis of cancer.

_____

c. Risk for body image disturbance related to loss of body part.

_____

13. Identify any additional nursing diagnoses for Mrs. Marshall.

_____

_____

14. *Word jumble:* Unscramble the following words. Then unscramble the circled letters to complete the sentence: The most frequent site of breast cancer in women is the

_____

1. S G T (E) P A

2. T (A) S M (T) S I I

3. (F) A M B E N R (O) O D I A

4. O A (E) A R (L)

5. (P) N (I) E L P

6. I I N (C) A

7. C O A M Y G (N) T (S) E A I

Name: _____	*Date:* _____
Course: _____	*Instructor:* _____

Student Lab Sheet: Assessing the Breasts

Health History

Biographical data:

Current health status: symptom analysis (PQRST):

- Lump or mass
- Pain or tenderness
- Nipple discharge

Past health history:

- Childhood illnesses
- Hospitalizations
- Surgeries
- Serious injuries/chronic illness
- Immunizations
- Allergies (food, drugs, environmental)
- Medications (prescribed and OTC)
- Recent travel/military service

Family history:

Review of systems:

- General health status
- HEENT
- Respiratory
- Cardiovascular
- Gastrointestinal
- Genitourinary
- Musculoskeletal
- Neurological
- Endocrine
- Lymphatic/hematological

Psychosocial profile:

- Health practices and beliefs/self-care activities
- Typical day
- Nutritional patterns (24-hour recall)
- Activity/exercise patterns
- Recreation, pets, hobbies
- Sleep/rest patterns
- Personal habits (tobacco, alcohol, caffeine, and drugs)
- Occupational health patterns
- Socioeconomic status
- Environmental health patterns
- Roles, relationships, self-concept
- Cultural/religious influences
- Family roles/relationships
- Sexuality patterns
- Social supports
- Stress/coping

Physical Assessment

General survey:

- Vital signs
- Height
- Weight

Head-to-toe scan:

Integumentary
- HEENT
- Respiratory
- Cardiovascular
- Abdomen
- Genitourinary
- Musculoskeletal
- Neurological

Assessing the Breasts

Area/Physical Assessment Skill	Assessment	Normal Findings Developmental/Cultural Variations	Student's Findings
Inspection	**Positions: sitting with arms at side, arms over head, hands on hips, or leaning forward, or supine with pillow under shoulder of breast being examined**		NO ABNORMAL MASSES
Breasts	Assess size, shape, symmetry, color. Note visible masses, lesions, edema, and venous pattern **Have client press hands together or press hands on hips to check for dimpling or retraction** Note dominant side	Breasts lobular, symmetrical, color consistent with body color. No masses, lesions, edema, dimpling, retraction, or orange peel skin May normally be slightly asymmetrical. Adolescent girls may have asymmetrical breasts as they go through puberty. Adolescent boys may have gynecomastia. During pregnancy, breasts enlarge, venous pattern increases, and areola and nipple darken in color. Postmenopausal breasts lose elasticity and are more pendulous	SYMMETRICAL, COLOR CONSISTANT, NO ABNORMAL MASSES, SLIGHT TENDERNESS TO TOUCH, NO LESIONS OR EDEMA

Nipple and areola	Note color, shape, symmetry, inversion/eversion, discharge, masses, lesions, and direction of nipples Inspect for supernumerary nipples	Nipples and areola symmetrical, round, and darker than breast tissue. Color lighter in fair-skinned and darker in dark-skinned women. No masses, lesions, or discharge. Spontaneous discharge normal during pregnancy and lactation. Symmetrical nipple direction, usually lateral and upward. Nipples may be everted, flat, or inverted, but should be symmetrical. No supernumerary nipples	COLOR FAIR SKINNED, NIPPLES DARKER, SYMMETRICAL NIPPLES SHOULD BE SYMMETRICAL
Axilla	Note color, lesions, masses, and hair distribution	Skin intact, no lesions or rashes. Hair growth appropriate for client's age and sex	NO LESIONS / RASH MINIMAL HAIR GROWTH
Palpation	**Use finger pads of three middle fingers, making small circles with light, medium, and deep pressure**		
Breasts	**Palpate from clavicle to sixth to seventh ICS and from sternum to midaxillary line. Use vertical strip, pie wedge, or circular method** Note texture, consistency, tenderness, or masses	Breast consistency depends on a woman's developmental stage Premenopausal breast more firm and elastic; breasts during pregnancy and lactation firm and tender; postmenopausal breasts less firm and elastic with stringy ducts Nontender, but may be tender and nodular premenstrually No masses or lesions	BREAST FIRM & ELASTIC MILD TENDERNESS

Assessing the Breasts (Continued)

Area/Physical Assessment Skill	Assessment	Normal Findings Developmental/Cultural Variations	Student's Findings
Nipple and areola	Note elasticity, discharge, or tenderness **Unless pregnant or lactating, spontaneous discharge is abnormal and warrants follow-up**	Nipple elastic, nontender, no discharge or white sebaceous secretion with nipple compression Pregnant or lactating women may have milky discharge	NIPPLE NON TENDER, NO DISCHARGE
Axilla and clavicular nodes: Central Anterior Posterior Lateral Epitrochlear Supraclavicular Infraclavicular	Note palpable nodes, location, tenderness, size, shape, consistency, mobility, borders, and temperature	Lymph nodes nonpalpable, nontender	NO TENDERNESS

Pertinent Health History Findings:

Pertinent Physical Assessment Findings:

Nursing Diagnoses (actual or potential) with Clustered Data:

Name: _____   Date: _____

Course: _____   Instructor: _____

Self-Evaluation Exercise

Breast Assessment	YES	NO	NEED MORE PRACTICE
1. Applies knowledge of anatomy and physiology of the breast in performing an assessment of the breast			
2. Applies growth and development principles as applicable to the breast			
3. Considers cultural variations as indicated when performing a breast assessment			
4. Gathers all equipment necessary to perform a breast assessment			
5. Obtains history specific to assessment of the breast			
6. Performs a physical assessment of the breast, including • General survey and head-to-toe scan • Inspection • Palpation			
7. Documents breast assessment findings			
8. Identifies normal/abnormal findings			
9. Clusters pertinent subjective/objective data			
10. Identifies actual/potential health problems and states them as nursing diagnoses with supporting data			

Chapter 15

Assessing the Abdomen

Name: _____	Date: _____
Course: _____	Instructor: _____

1. Anatomy review: Label the following structures.

   - Liver
   - Gallbladder
   - Small intestine
   - Ascending colon
   - Transverse colon
   - Descending colon
   - Stomach
   - Appendix
   - Urinary bladder
   - Spleen

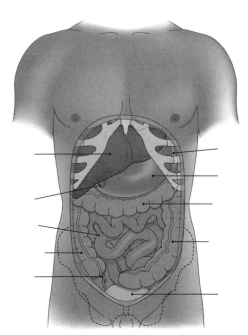

2. Match the structure in the first column to its description in the second column.

Structure	Description
1. Esophagus B	a. Primary site for digestion
2. Pancreas D	b. Muscular tube that connects mouth to stomach
3. Small intestines A	c. Stores bile
4. Gallbladder C	d. Secretes insulin, glucagons, and digestive enzymes
5. Appendix F	e. Connects small and large intestines
6. Ileocecal valve E	f. Common site of infection
7. Liver G	g. Reabsorbs water

8. Large intestines _g_   h. Produce saliva and amylase

9. Stomach _i_   i. Churns food and secretes intrinsic factor and hydrochloric acid

10. Salivary glands _h_   j. Primary function is metabolism and detoxification

3. Place the following structures in the correct quadrants.

- Liver __RIGHT UPPER QUAD__

- Gallbladder __RIGH UPPER QUAD__

- Pancreas __RIGHT UPPER QUAD__

- Stomach __LEFT UPPER QUAD__

- Spleen __LEFT UPPER QUAT__

- Cecum __RIGHT LOWER QUAD__

- Appendix __RIGHT LOWER QUAD__

- Sigmoid colon __LEFT LOWER QUAD__

- Transverse colon __RIGHT UPPER QUAD , RIGHT LOWER & LEFT UPPER__

- Ascending colon __RIGHT UPPER QUAD__

- Descending colon __LEFT UPPER & LEFT LOWER__

4. Match the origin of pain in the first column to the referred area of pain in the second column.

Origin of Pain   **Referred Area of Pain**

1. Ruptured spleen _c_   a. Scapula

2. Cholecystitis _a_   b. Flank and thighs

3. Abdominal aortic aneurysm _d_   c. Shoulder

4. Early appendicitis _e_   d. Low back

5. Renal problems _b_   e. Umbilical area

5. Lou Walker, age 63, had a colon resection 3 days ago. He is NPO and has a nasogastric tube connected to low suction. You begin his abdominal assessment with inspection. What three movements should you look for when inspecting the abdomen?
   __RESPIRATIONS , PERISTALSIS & PULSATIONS__

6. After inspecting Mr. Walker's abdomen, you auscultate it. What is the rationale for performing auscultation before palpating the abdomen?
   __PALPATATION COULD ALTER BOWEL SOUNDS__

7. You have trouble auscultating Mr. Walker's bowel sounds. How long should you auscultate before charting that bowel sounds are absent?
   __5 MIN.__

8. Before charting that Mr. Walker has absent bowel sounds, listen over the ileocecal valve. Where is this site located, and what is the rationale for listening over it?

ICL - Right lower

RATIONALE: ACTIVE SITE CONNECTS SMALL INTESTINE

9. Mr. Walker's abdomen is distended, and his bowel sounds are hypoactive. How do you explain these findings?

EFFECTS OF ANESTHESIA, ABDOMINAL SURGERY, & DECREASE MOBILITY

10. Name two causes for hypoactive or absent bowel sounds.

PAIN MEDS & IMMOBILITY

11. Name two causes of hyperactive bowel sounds.

DIARRHEA & EARLY OBSTRUCTION.

12. Bill Dwyer, age 56, has been diagnosed with early cirrhosis. Abdominal assessment includes percussion of the liver for size. What test would help you locate the lower border of the liver?

SCRATCH TEST

13. What percussion sound would you expect to elicit over the liver?

DULLNESS

14. Mr. Dwyer's liver measures 14 cm at the midclavicular line. What is the normal liver size at the midclavicular line?

6-12 CM

15. Brian Duffy, a 20-year-old college student, comes to the ED after being injured during a lacrosse game. He presents with left upper quadrant pain. You assess for splenic enlargement and find that his spleen is palpable in the left upper quadrant at the costal margin. Is this a normal finding? Why or why not?

NO THE SPLEEN NEEDS TO BE QUITE LARGE TO BE PALPABLE

16. You assess Brian's spleen further through percussion. Where do you percuss to locate the spleen?

MIDAXILLARY LINE

17. Although your assessment focuses on the abdomen, all systems are related. What assessment findings (subjective or objective) show the relationship between the abdomen and other systems?

WEIGHT CHANGES, SKIN, HAIR & NAILS, THYROID DISEASE, VISION, BREATHING, INSPECT FACIAL EXPRESSION, HAIR SKIN EP.

Name: _____	*Date:* _____
Course: _____	*Instructor:* _____

Abnormal Case Study: Larry Petroski

Larry Petroski, age 25, is admitted to the ED with complaints of nausea, vomiting, and abdominal pain. He is bent over and walking slowly. He states, "I think I have food poisoning." Because his problem is acute, you perform a focused health history.

Health History

Chief complaint:

"I think I have food poisoning."

Symptom analysis:

P—Standing up makes pain worse, and nothing makes it better.

Q—Describes pain as "sharp and constant."

R—Client states, "I'm having such pain in my belly." Says that pain was initially around umbilical area, then shifted to right lower quadrant. Denies any radiation.

S—States pain is 10 on the 0-to-10 scale.

T—States that pain started acutely around 10 a.m. and has progressively worsened. He was brought to ED at 1 p.m.

Current health history:

Client states, "I am always healthy and never had any problems with my belly before."

Past health history:

- This is client's first hospital admission.
- No previous health problems.
- Takes no medications.

Family history:

- Mother died of lung cancer.
- Father alive and well with no health problems.
- No siblings.

Psychosocial profile:

- *Nutritional patterns:* States that he was able to eat his usual breakfast (cereal and milk) at 8 a.m. Abdominal pain started at 10 a.m., then nausea and vomiting at 10:30 a.m. States that he thinks he has food poisoning.
- *Recreation/hobbies:* Enjoys riding his snowmobile and motorcycle and taking long walks along beach with his wife.
- *Occupational health patterns:* Works as an auto mechanic.
- *Environmental health patterns:* Lives in a suburban city in a one-story house near the ocean.
- *Roles/relationships:* Lives with his wife and daughter and spends a great deal of time with daughter. Is active in local church.

In gastroenteritis, nausea and vomiting occur before onset of abdominal pain; in appendicitis, the opposite occurs.

Physical Assessment

- *General appearance:* Appears in obvious distress with his body bent over and his arms covering his abdomen.
- *Vital signs:* Temperature 37.9°C; pulse 89 beats/min; respirations 24/min; BP 139/70 mm Hg.
- *Mental status:* Alert and oriented × 4.
- *Urine:* Yellow and without sediment.
- *Leg edema:* No edema present throughout the body.

- *Inspection:*
- Abdomen uniformly tan in color.
- No striae, bruises, or hernias noted; umbilicus centered.
- Abdomen flat and symmetrical without distention.

- No aortic pulsations; peristalsis noted.
- Abdominal respiratory pattern shallow with increased respiratory rate.

18. Because Mr. Petroski has an abdominal problem, how would you explain the shallow respiratory pattern and increase in respiratory rate?

_____

_____

Auscultation:
- Hypoactive bowel sounds in all four quadrants.
- No bruits, friction rubs, or venous hums.

Percussion:
- Liver span 4.0.
- Unable to percuss bladder or spleen.
- Negative costovertebral angle tenderness.

Palpation:
- Light and deep palpation could not be performed on Mr. Petroski because of abdominal pain. Consequently, many of the palpation tests were limited to the essential test, which included the following results:

- Muscle guarding in the right lower quadrant.
- Tenderness in the right lower quadrant.

Additional assessment data:
- Rebound tenderness at McBurney's point.
- Positive iliopsoas muscle test.
- Positive obturator muscle test.
- Positive cutaneous hypersensitivity in right lower quadrant.
- Positive Rovsing's sign.

19. Mr. Petroski ate breakfast at 8 a.m. What is the importance of identifying the time he last ate?

_____

_____

20. What additional question should you ask Mr. Petroski if he is scheduled for surgery or will be receiving any medication?

_____

_____

21. Which of Mr. Petroski's vital signs are abnormal, and what are the causes of these variations?

_____

_____

22. What physical findings indicate appendicitis?

_____

_____

_____

23. Mr. Petroski was diagnosed as having appendicitis, and he was scheduled for emergency surgery. Cluster the supporting data for the following nursing diagnoses for him:

    a. Pain: Acute related to obstruction of the appendix with inflammation.

    _____

    b. Alteration in comfort: nausea and vomiting related to stimulation of vomiting center from pain.

    _____

    c. Potential for fluid volume defect related to nausea and vomiting.

    _____

24. Your first priority nursing diagnosis is pain: acute related to obstruction of the appendix with inflammation. Select some appropriate preoperative nursing actions.

    _____

    _____

25. One complication of appendicitis is peritonitis. What data should you obtain to ascertain if Mr. Petroski's appendix has ruptured?

    _____

    _____

26. Identify any additional nursing diagnoses for this client.

    _____

    _____

27. *Word jumble:* Unscramble the following words. Then unscramble the circled letter to complete the sentence: The area of tenderness in acute appendicitis is

_____

   1. Ⓡ L V I E

   2. S Ⓟ T L A S I E R I S

   3. E R A Ⓣ Ⓢ I

   4. L E A Ⓜ E N

   5. Ⓤ F L S A T

   6. Y H Ⓒ E M

   7. R O G B Ⓨ I M R O Ⓑ

   8. S I C T E A S

   9. H A Ⓔ R I D A R

  10. T M I Ⓞ C A S A T Ⓝ

  11. E Ⓝ L P S E

  12. H S Ⓘ C R O R I S

Name: _____ Date: _____

Course: _____ Instructor: _____

Student Lab Sheet: Assessing the Abdomen

Health History

Biographical data:

Current health status: symptom analysis (PQRST):

- Elimination pattern: frequency, color, and consistency of stool.
- Abdominal pain.
- Nausea and vomiting.
- Weight changes.
- Appetite.

Past health history:

- Childhood illnesses
- Hospitalizations
- Surgeries
- Serious injuries/chronic illness
- Immunizations
- Allergies (food, drugs, environmental)
- Medications (prescribed and OTC)
- Recent travel/military service

Family history:

Review of systems:

- General health status
- HEENT
- Respiratory
- Cardiovascular
- Genitourinary
- Musculoskeletal
- Neurological
- Endocrine
- Lymphatic/hematological

Psychosocial profile:

- Health practices and beliefs/self-care activities
- Typical day
- Nutritional patterns (24-hour recall)
- Activity/exercise patterns
- Recreation, pets, hobbies
- Sleep/rest patterns
- Personal habits (tobacco, alcohol, caffeine, and drugs)
- Occupational health patterns
- Socioeconomic status
- Environmental health patterns
- Roles, relationships, self-concept
- Cultural/religious influences
- Family roles/relationships
- Sexuality patterns
- Social supports
- Stress/coping

Physical Assessment

General survey:

- Vital signs
- Height
- Weight

Head-to-toe scan:

- General health status
- Integumentary
- HEENT
- Respiratory
- Cardiovascular
- Genitourinary
- Musculoskeletal
- Neurological

Assessing the Abdomen

Area/Physical Assessment Skill	Assessment	Normal Findings Developmental/Cultural Variations	Student's Findings
Inspection	**Inspect from side and foot of bed. Have client void before exam** **Position: supine**		
Abdomen	Note size, shape, and symmetry of abdomen	Skin color consistent or slightly lighter than exposed areas. No lesions, striae, superficial veins, scars, rashes, or discoloration. Hair distribution appropriate for client's age and gender	
	Note condition of skin, color, lesions, scars, striae, superficial veins, and hair distribution		
	Note abdominal movements: respiratory, pulsation, and peristalsis	Abdomen flat or slightly rounded and symmetrical, no bulges or hernias	
	Note position, contour, color, and herniation of umbilicus	Positive respiratory movements, slight pulsation noted in epigastric region, no peristaltic waves	
	Have client raise head off bed, then check for bulges (hernias)	Umbilicus midline, inverted, no discoloration or discharge	
		Pregnant client may have increased pigmentation at midline (linea nigra), striae, diastasis recti, and upward and outward displacement of umbilicus	
		Children also may have diastasis recti	

Auscultation	**Always auscultate before palpating. Palpation may after bowel sounds** **Use diaphragm of stethoscope for bowel sounds and friction rubs** **Use bell for vascular sounds**	
Abdomen Liver Arteries	Listen for bowel sounds in each quadrant Listen for at least 5 minutes before saying bowel sounds are absent **If having difficulty hearing bowel sounds, listen over ileocecal valve to right of umbilicus in right lower quadrant** Use scratch test to locate inferior edge of liver Auscultate for bruits over aorta, renal, iliac, and femoral arteries If indicated, auscultate for venous hum over liver If indicated, auscultate for friction rubs over organs	Soft, medium-pitched bowel sounds every 5–15 seconds in all four quadrants No borborygmi, bruits, hums, or rubs Lower edge of liver located at costal margin by scratch test
Percussion	**Use indirect (mediate) percussion in all four quadrants**	

Assessing the Abdomen (Continued)

Area/Physical Assessment Skill	Assessment	Normal Findings Developmental/Cultural Variations	Student's Findings
Abdominal organs (liver, gallbladder, spleen, kidneys)	Note areas of tympany, dullness, or tenderness	Tympany in all four quadrants, dullness over organs. Liver 6–12 cm at right midclavicular line; 4–8 cm at the midsternal line	
	Measure liver size at the right midclavicular line. If enlarged, measure at midsternal line	Spleenic dullness 9th, 10th, 11th ribs at right midaxillary line, < 7cm	
	Locate gastric bubble over stomach	Organs nontender	
	Locate splenic dullness at left midaxillary line		
	If ascites, percuss for shifting dullness		
	If indicated, use fist (blunt) percussion to assess for organ (liver or gallbladder) tenderness. Check for kidney tenderness at posterior costovertebral angle		
	Percuss tender areas last		
Palpation	**Begin with light palpation, then to deep, bimanual palpation in all four quadrants**		
	If client tenses (voluntary guarding), have him or her slightly flex knees, or let client hold your hand as you palpate		
Aorta	Note size and pulsation	Aorta 2.5 cm. slight pulsation palpable. No diffusion	

Abdominal organs	Use light palpation to identify surface characteristics, tenderness, muscular resistance, and turgor and to put client at ease. Assess umbilicus for bulges or nodules ***Do not palpate abdomen if client has Wilms's tumor, large diffuse pulsations, or history of organ transplant*** Use deep palpation with bimanual technique to palpate organs (liver, spleen, kidneys) and masses. Note tenderness, consistency, pulsations, and enlarged organs. Palpate aorta, noting pulsation, size, and diffusion If indicated, assess for rebound tenderness at McBurney's point, the iliopsoas test, and the obturator test If fluid, test for fluid wave test Use ballottement to assess fetal position or masses Test abdominal reflexes by lightly stroking each quadrant toward the umbilicus If possible gallbladder disease, assess Murphy's sign If possible splenic injury or rupture, assess Kehr's and balance signs	Abdomen soft, nontender, no masses, positive skin turgor, and negative umbilical bulges Liver nonpalpable or liver's edge palpable at costal margin, firm, smooth, and nontender Spleen nontender, nonpalpable Negative rebound Kidneys usually nonpalpable. Right kidney may be palpable in thin woman Positive slight aortic pulsation, no diffusion, aorta 2.5 cm Positive abdominal reflexes
Inguinal lymph nodes	Use light palpation; palpate horizontal and vertical inguinal nodes. Note size, shape, consistency, tenderness, and mobility	Inguinal nodes nonpalpable, nontender

Pertinent Health History Findings:

Pertinent Physical Assessment Findings:

Nursing Diagnoses (actual or potential) with Clustered Data:

Name: _____   Date: _____

Course: _____   Instructor: _____

Self-Evaluation Exercise

Abdominal Assessment	YES	NO	NEED MORE PRACTICE
1. Applies knowledge of anatomy and physiology of the abdomen in performing an assessment of the abdomen			
2. Applies growth and development principles as applicable to the abdomen			
3. Considers cultural variations as indicated when performing an abdominal assessment			
4. Gathers all equipment necessary to perform an abdominal assessment			
5. Obtains history specific to assessment of the abdomen			
6. Perform a physical assessment of the abdomen, including • General survey and head-to-toe scan • Inspection • Auscultation • Percussion • Palpation			
7. Documents abdominal assessment findings			
8. Identifies normal/abnormal findings			
9. Clusters pertinent subjective/objective data			
10. Identifies actual/potential health problems and states them as nursing diagnoses with supporting data			

Name: _____	*Date:* _____
Course: _____	*Instructor:* _____

Student Lab Sheet: Assessing the Female Genitourinary System

Health History

Biographical data:

Current health status: symptom analysis (PQRST):

- Vaginal discharge
- Pain
- Lumps/masses
- Dysmenorrhea
- Amenorrhea
- Urinary symptoms

Past health history:

- Childhood illnesses
- Hospitalizations
- Surgeries
- Serious injuries/chronic illness
- Immunizations
- Allergies (food, drugs, environmental)
- Medications (prescribed and OTC)
- Recent travel/military service

Family history:

Review of systems:

- General health status
- HEENT
- Respiratory
- Cardiovascular
- Gastrointestinal
- Musculoskeletal
- Neurological
- Endocrine
- Lymphatic/hematological

Psychosocial profile:

- Health practices and beliefs/self-care activities
- Typical day
- Nutritional patterns (24-hour recall)
- Activity/exercise patterns
- Recreation, pets, hobbies
- Sleep/rest patterns
- Personal habits (tobacco, alcohol, caffeine, and drugs)
- Occupational health patterns
- Socioeconomic status
- Environmental health patterns
- Roles, relationships, self-concept
- Cultural/religious influences
- Family roles/relationships
- Sexuality patterns
- Social supports
- Stress/coping

Physical Assessment

General survey:

- Vital signs
- Height
- Weight

Head-to-toe scan:

- General health status
- Integumentary
- HEENT
- Respiratory
- Cardiovascular
- Abdominal
- Musculoskeletal
- Neurological

Assessing the Female Genitourinary System

Area/Physical Assessment Skill	Assessment	Normal Findings Developmental/Cultural Variations	Student's Findings
Inspection	**Position:** lithotomy **Maintain universal precautions, wear gloves**		
External genitalia	**Have client void before exam**		
Labia majora Labia minora Clitoris Urethra Vaginal orifice Skene's glands Bartholin's glands Perineum	Note color, hair distribution, condition of skin, swelling, lesions, polyps, discharge, odor, prolapse, or pubic pediculosis	External genitalia intact, pink, and moist; color depends on client's pigmentation. Hair distribution depends on age and development of client No lesions, edema, discharge, odor, or prolapse (bladder, uterus, or rectum) Normal cervical discharge depends on menstrual cycle: clear and stretchy before ovulation, white and opaque after ovulation, bloody during menstruation	
Rectal area	Note condition of skin, inflammation, rashes, excoriation, rectal prolapse, external hemorrhoids, polyps, lesions, fissures, bleeding, and discharge	Rectal area intact, no inflammation, lesions, prolapse, hemorrhoids, discharge, or bleeding	

Assessment	Procedure	Normal Findings
Pelvic exam with speculum: Cervix Vaginal walls	Use warm speculum Note color, lesions, discharge, bleeding, position, size, shape and symmetry, shape and patency of os Obtain specimens as indicated Inspect vaginal walls while withdrawing speculum	Cervix round, midline, pink, no lesions or discharge, os is slit in parous female, round and closed in nulliparous female. Bluish color seen with pregnancy, paler color seen in postmenopausal women Vaginal walls pink with rugae, no lesions
Palpation	**Lubricate index and middle fingers of gloved hand. Perform vaginal exam first, then speculum exam, bimanual exam, and rectovaginal exam**	
Skene's glands, Bartholin's glands	Usually performed before speculum insertion Insert index finger into vagina with finger pad upward, and milk urethra and Skene's gland Note any masses, swelling, discharge, or tenderness	Area smooth; no swelling, masses, or tenderness
Vaginal walls	Note texture, swelling, lesions, or tenderness	Vaginal wall rugae: no swelling, lesions, nodules, or tenderness. Less rugae in postmenopausal women
Perineum	Assess tone and texture	Perineum smooth, firm in the multiparous woman, thinner in parous woman
Cervix	Note size, shape, consistency, position, mobility, or tenderness	Cervix round, smooth, firm, midline, mobile, and nontender Cervix smaller in older women Cervix softer and enlarged during pregnancy

Assessing the Female Genitourinary System (*Continued*)

Area/Physical Assessment Skill	Assessment	Normal Findings Developmental/Cultural Variations	Student's Findings
Uterus	Note size, shape, symmetry, position, masses, or tenderness	Uterus midline, may be anteflexed or anteverted, midplane, retroflexed, or retroverted. Pear-shaped, size increases with pregnancy, firm, mobile, slightly tender. No masses	
Ovaries	Note size, shape, symmetry, or tenderness	Ovaries usually nonpalpable; if palpable, almond-shaped, firm, smooth, about $3 \times 2 \times 1$ cm, mobile, sensitive to palpation. Ovaries not palpable in postmenopausal women or prepubertal girls	
Anus and rectum	***Change gloves before rectovaginal exam to prevent cross-contamination*** Perform rectal exam and note sphincter tone, pain, tenderness, nodules, lesions, masses, hemorrhoids, polyps, or bleeding Note color of stool; **test for occult blood**	Positive sphincter tone; nontender; no masses, polyps, lesions, hemorrhoids, or bleeding Stool brown, negative for occult blood	

Pertinent Health History Findings:

_____

Pertinent Physical Findings:

_____

Nursing Diagnoses (actual or potential) with Clustered Data:

_____

Name: _____	Date: _____
Course: _____	Instructor: _____

Self-Evaluation Exercise

Female Genitourinary System	YES	NO	NEED MORE PRACTICE
1. Applies knowledge of anatomy and physiology of the female genitourinary system in performing an assessment of the female genitourinary system			
2. Applies growth and development principles as applicable to the female genitourinary system			
3. Considers cultural variations as indicated when performing a female genitourinary assessment			
4. Gathers all equipment necessary to perform a female genitourinary assessment			
5. Obtains history specific to assessment of the female genitourinary system			
6. Performs a physical assessment of the female genitourinary system, including • General survey and head-to-toe scan • Inspection • Palpation • Pelvic exam			
7. Documents female genitourinary assessment findings.			
8. Identifies normal/abnormal findings			
9. Clusters pertinent subjective/objective data			
10. Identifies actual/potential health problems and states them as nursing diagnoses with supporting data			

Name: _____ Date: _____

Course: _____ Instructor: _____

Abnormal Case Study: Mike Samuels

Mike Samuels is a 22-year-old college junior. He is on the football team, lives in a residence hall, and does not own a car. He has had six girlfriends during his 3 years at college and has been sexually active with each. Since age 16, he has had gonorrhea once and chlamydia once. He admits that he uses condoms only occasionally. He presents to the clinic saying, "One of my old girlfriends just called me to say that she had a positive HIV test and that I should get checked out."

Health History

Chief complaint:

"One of my old girlfriends just called me to say that she had a positive HIV test and that I should get checked out."

Current health status: Denies any physical symptoms.

Past health history:

- Had an HIV test 2 years ago as part of his athletic physical. Test results were negative for syphilis and HIV.
- Gonorrhea 5 years ago, treated; return test was negative.
- Chlamydia 3 years ago, treated; did not return for retesting.

9. In this sensitive situation, how would you proceed with the evaluation?

_____

_____

_____

_____

10. From Mr. Samuels's history, identify factors that increase his risk for sexually transmitted diseases (STDs).

_____

_____

11. There are no obvious signs or symptoms to suggest HIV infection. Based on the inspection findings what other problem would you suspect?

_____

12. Considering Mr. Samuels's assessment findings, what areas should you address for client education?

_____

_____

Psychosocial profile:

- *Nutritional patterns:* Usually has healthy appetite, although hasn't been hungry since previous girlfriend contacted him about HIV.
- *Activity/exercise patterns:* Plays on football team.
- *Recreation/hobbies:* No time for hobbies; enjoys dating in spare time, which is usually evenings after studying.
- *Sleep/rest patterns:* Sleeps 5 hours/night.
- *Personal habits:* Smokes marijuana at least once a week, drinks "a lot" of alcohol on the weekends when there is no football game or after the game. Has never used cocaine, barbiturates, narcotics, amphetamines, or intravenous drugs. Has never had a blood transfusion. Has had multiple female sex partners. Has never had sex with another man. Has not knowingly had sex with a prostitute. Engages in sex at least three times a week; occasionally uses condoms.
- *Occupational health patterns:* Student who attends class regularly.
- *Environmental health patterns:* Lives in college residence hall with one roommate. All of his peers have several female friends.

Physical Assessment

- *General appearance:* Healthy 22-year-old man; 6 feet, 1 inch and 195 lb; keeps head down and makes minimal eye contact; appears anxious.
- *Vital signs:* Normal.
- *Integumentary:*
- No skin lesions on head, torso, or extremities.
- Hair evenly distributed; no alopecia.
- No parasites.
- *HEENT:*
- Oropharynx is pink and moist without lesions.
- No cervical lymphadenopathy.

Penis:

- No discharge from penis; multiple wartlike lesions on shaft.
- No masses felt.
- No discharge from urethral meatus.

Scrotum:

- Scrotal skin intact without swelling or lesions. Left is lower than right.
- No inguinal bulges.
- Testicles are firm, nontender, and smooth. Epididymis is insensitive to pressure.

Inguinal area:

- No lymphadenopathy; no palpable masses in inguinal canals bilaterally.

13. Cluster the supporting data for the following nursing diagnoses.

    a. Altered health maintenance related to risky behavior and knowledge deficit of STDs.

    _____

    _____

    b. Risk for infection related to lack of knowledge of disease transmission.

    _____

    _____

    c. Risk for infection transmission related to lack of knowledge of disease transmission.

    _____

    _____

14. Identify any additional nursing diagnoses for Mr. Samuels.

_____

_____

15. *Word search:* Find the following words in the puzzle: ejaculate, erection, hernia, penis, prostate, scrotum, semen, sperm, testes, urethra.

```
S  N  O  I  T  C  E  R  E  P
E  C  E  J  A  C  U  T  A  E
H  E  R  N  I  A  S  E  M  N
S  C  R  O  T  U  M  A  C  I
P  R  O  S  T  A  T  E  P  S
E  J  A  C  U  L  A  T  E  U
R  I  N  S  S  E  M  E  N  L
M  U  R  E  T  H  R  A  I  A
P  E  R  S  S  E  T  S  E  T
H  E  R  N  I  S  P  E  R  E
```

Name: _____   Date: _____

Course: _____   Instructor: _____

Student Lab Sheet: Assessing the Male Genitourinary System

Health History

Biographical data:

Current health status: symptom analysis (PQRST):

- Pain
- Lesions
- Discharge
- Swelling
- Urinary symptoms
- Erectile dysfunction

Past health history:

- Childhood illnesses
- Hospitalizations
- Surgeries
- Serious injuries/chronic illness
- Immunizations
- Allergies (food, drugs, environmental)
- Medications (prescribed and OTC)
- Recent travel/military service

Family history:

Review of systems:

- General health status
- HEENT
- Respiratory
- Cardiovascular
- Gastrointestinal
- Musculoskeletal
- Neurological
- Endocrine
- Lymphatic/hematological

Psychosocial profile:

- Health practices and beliefs/self-care activities
- Typical day
- Nutritional patterns (24-hour recall)
- Activity/exercise patterns
- Recreation, pets, hobbies
- Sleep/rest patterns
- Personal habits (tobacco, alcohol, caffeine, and drugs)
- Occupational health patterns
- Socioeconomic status
- Environmental health patterns
- Roles, relationships, self-concept
- Cultural/religious influences
- Family roles/relationships
- Sexuality patterns
- Social supports
- Stress/coping

Physical Assessment

General survey:

- Vital signs
- Height
- Weight

Head-to-toe scan:

- General health status
- Integumentary
- HEENT
- Respiratory
- Cardiovascular
- Abdominal
- Musculoskeletal
- Neurological

Assessing the Male Genitourinary System

Area/Physical Assessment Skill	Assessment	Normal Findings Developmental/Cultural Variations	Student's Findings
Inspection	**Position:** standing, have client void before exam.		
Penis	Inspect dorsal, lateral, and ventral sides	Skin intact, color pink to light brown in whites, light to dark brown in blacks, no lesions or discharge.	
	Note condition and color of skin, lesions, and discharge	Urinary meatus midline at tip of glans, foreskin retracts easily	
	Note size in relation to physical development and age		
	Note position of urinary meatus		
	Note presence of foreskin or circumcised. If uncircumcised, retract foreskin, note ease of retraction and presence of lesions		
Scrotum	Note color, hair distribution, lesions, swelling, size, and position. Note pubic pediculosis	Skin color darker than rest of body. Hair distribution appropriate for age of client	
		Testes hang freely. Left testis slightly lower than right	
		No lesions, pediculosis	
Inguinal area	Note condition of skin, bulges	Skin intact, no bulges, no palpable lymph nodes	
	Have client bear down and inspect again for any bulges		
	Note enlarged lymph nodes		

Rectal area	Note condition of skin, inflammation, rashes, excoriation, rectal prolapse, external hemorrhoids, polyps, lesions, fissures, bleeding, or discharge	Rectal area intact, no inflammation, lesions, prolapse, hemorrhoids, discharge, or bleeding
Palpation	Maintain universal precautions, wear gloves	
Penis	Note consistency, tenderness, induration, masses, or nodules Use thumb and two fingers to palpate shaft	Nonerect penis soft, nontender, no nodules
Scrotum, testes, and epididymis	Use thumb and two fingers to palpate surface characteristics of scrotum. Note size, shape, consistency, mobility, masses, nodules, and tenderness of testes Palpate epididymis and vas deferens on the posterolateral surface, noting swelling or nodules **Transilluminate any lumps, nodules, or edematous areas**	Scrotal skin rough without lesions. Testes rubbery, round, movable, smooth, 2 cm × 5 cm in size, slightly tender with compression The ridge of epididymis noted and vas deferens smooth and movable. No swelling or nodules
Inguinal area	Palpate for inguinal and femoral hernias or masses. **Have client bear down or cough as you palpate for a bulge or hernia** Palpate lymph nodes, horizontal and vertical chain. Note enlargement and tenderness	No inguinal or femoral hernias or masses. No palpable lymph nodes

Assessing the Male Genitourinary System (*Continued*)

Area/Physical Assessment Skill	Assessment	Normal Findings Developmental/Cultural Variations	Student's Findings
Anus and rectum	**Position:** have client bend over exam table or lie on side. Note sphincter tone, pain, tenderness, nodules, lesions, masses, hemorrhoids, polyps, or bleeding Note color of stool; **test for occult blood**	Positive sphincter tone, nontender, no masses, polyps, lesions, hemorrhoids, or bleeding Stool brown; negative for occult blood	
Prostate	Note size, shape, symmetry, mobility, consistency, nodules, or tenderness	Prostate walnut shape and size, smooth, rubbery, nontender	
Auscultation	If scrotal mass detected, auscultate over scrotum for bowel sounds. If present, sign of indirect inguinal hernia	No bowel sounds	

Pertinent Health History Findings:

Pertinent Physical Assessment Findings:

Nursing Diagnoses (actual or potential) with Clustered Data:

Name: _____   Date: _____

Course: _____   Instructor: _____

Self-Evaluation Exercise

Male Genitourinary System	YES	NO	NEED MORE PRACTICE
1. Applies knowledge of anatomy and physiology of the male genitourinary system in performing an assessment of the male genitourinary system			
2. Applies growth and development principles as applicable to the male genitourinary system			
3. Considers cultural variations as indicated when performing a male genitourinary assessment			
4. Gathers all equipment necessary to perform a male genitourinary assessment			
5. Obtains history specific to assessment of the male genitourinary system			
6. Performs a physical assessment of the male genitourinary system, including • General survey and head-to-toe scan • Inspection • Palpation • Auscultation • Digital rectal exam			
7. Documents male genitourinary assessment findings			
8. Identifies normal/abnormal findings			
9. Clusters pertinent subjective/objective data			
10. Identifies actual/potential health problems and states them as nursing diagnoses with supporting data			

Chapter 18

Assessing the Musculoskeletal System

| Name: _____ | Date: _____ |
| Course: _____ | Instructor: _____ |

1. Match the structure in the first column to its description in the second column.

Structure	Description
1. Bursa *(e)*	a. Allows for upright position and movement; produces heat
2. Tendon *(c)*	b. Provides structure and support, produces red blood cells, and stores calcium
3. Ligament *(d)*	c. Connects muscles to bone
4. Cartilage *(g)*	d. Connects bone to bone
5. Joint *(F)*	e. Sac filled with synovial fluid that cushions and decreases stress to joints
6. Muscle *(a)*	f. Articulation of two adjacent bones or cartilage
7. Bone *(B)*	g. Cushions and absorbs shock

2. What type of synovial joint corresponds to each of the following joints?

   a. Knee HINGE

   b. Shoulder BALL & SOCKET

   c. Wrist CONDYLOID

   d. Spine GLIDING / PLANE

   e. Elbow HINGE BALL

   f. Hip BALL IN SOCKET

   g. Thumb SADDLE

3. Match the movement in the first column to its description in the second column.

Movement	Description
1. Extension (d)	a. Movement away from midline
2. Flexion (h)	b. Turning inward toward midline
3. Internal rotation (b)	c. Pulling in or backward
4. External rotation (l)	d. Straightening a joint angle
5. Protraction (m)	e. Turning palms up
6. Retraction (c)	f. Turning soles of feet inward
7. Pronation (j)	g. Circular movement
8. Supination (e)	h. Shortening a joint angle
9. Inversion (f)	i. Movement toward the midline
10. Eversion (k)	j. Turning palms down
11. Abduction (a)	k. Turning soles of feet outward
12. Adduction (i)	l. Turning outward away from midline
13. Circumduction (g)	m. Pushing out or forward

4. You are assessing Sarah Parker, a 15-year-old high school sophomore, for scoliosis. You begin by inspecting her spine. What position is best for this?

   STANDING & BENDING OVER IN ONE POSITION

5. As you inspect Sarah's spine, you first note the normal curves. What are the four normal curves of the spine?

   THORACIC, CERVICAL, LUMBAR, SACRAL

6. Name and describe the three spinal deformities that you should assess during the spinal examination.

   KYPHOSIS - ACCENTUATED THORACIC CURVE
   SCOLIOSIS - LATERAL DEVIATED SPINE
   LORDOSIS - ACCENTUATED LUMBAR CURVE

7. Your assessment of Sarah includes leg and arm length measurements. Describe the proper techniques to measure arm lengths and leg lengths.

   _____

   _____

8. You note that Sarah's right leg is 2 cm longer than her left leg. Name three findings (subjective or objective) that reflect the effect of the leg-length discrepancy.

   _____

   _____

9. You note that Sarah's right upper arm circumference is 1.5 cm greater than her left upper arm circumference. How might you account for this?

_____

10. Helen Janewsky, age 70, has degenerative joint disease (DJD) and is 2 days postoperative after a total right hip replacement. She is ambulating with her walker. You are assessing her gait. What six characteristics should you note?

_____

_____

11. Name four changes from normal that you would expect to see in Mrs. Janewsky's gait.

_____

_____

12. What changes in gait might indicate a balance problem?

_____

13. Considering Mrs. Janewsky's age, what spinal deformity might you expect to see?

_____

14. Because Mrs. Janewsky has DJD, you do a complete assessment of her other joints. Name six characteristics you should note during joint assessment.

_____

_____

15. You are assessing Mrs. Janewsky's muscle strength. Your findings include: +5 arms, +4 left leg, and +3 right leg. How would you interpret these findings?

_____

_____

16. Assessment of cerebellar function includes balance, coordination, and accuracy of movement. Name five ways to assess balance.

_____

_____

17. Name two ways to test coordination of upper and lower extremities.

_____

_____

18. Name two ways to test accuracy of movements.

_____

_____

19. Although your assessment focuses on the musculoskeletal system, all systems are related. What assessment findings (subjective or objective) show the relationship between the musculoskeletal system and other systems?

_____

_____

_____

Name: _____ Date: _____

Course: _____ Instructor: _____

Abnormal Case Study: Linda Chu

Linda Chu, a 62-year-old Asian woman, is admitted to the cardiac catheterization unit for a diagnostic procedure to assess coronary artery disease. She is scheduled for the procedure the next morning. She states that she is unable to lie flat for long periods because of chronic low back pain. Because this procedure can take a long time, you need to perform an assessment.

Health History

Chief complaint:

"My lower back hurts all the time."

Symptom analysis:

P—Pain to lower back when sitting or lying for extended periods.
Q—"Feels like a dull knife in my lower back. I usually get up and walk around to relieve it."
R—"It's my bones; they are getting old."
S—7 on a scale of 1 to 10.
T—Diagnosed with DJD 2 years ago, which has been getting progressively worse.

Current health status:

- Pain when sitting or lying for extended periods; 7 on a scale of 1 to 10.
- Stands at her job in a mill pulling cloth through a cutter.
- Takes 4 to 8 ibuprofen tablets (Advil) a day for pain relief.
- Takes lisinopril (Zestril), 5mg once a daily for HTN.

Past health history:

- Normal childhood illnesses.
- Appendectomy at age 8.
- Denies allergies.
- Denies blood transfusions or handicaps.

Family history:

- Family history of HTN.
- Family history of DJD.

Psychosocial profile:

- *Nutritional patterns:* Eats three balanced meals a day—meat, potatoes, and vegetable. Good milk intake.
- *Recreation/hobbies:* Knits and plays bingo when back isn't hurting too much to sit.
- *Occupational health patterns:* Cutter in a cloth mill. Heavy lifting and pulling are involved in this line of work.
- *Environmental health patterns:* Lives in a two-story home in the country.
- *Roles/relationships:* Lives with husband of 30 years. Has two daughters who visit often. Has not been sexually active for several years because of back problems.

Physical Assessment

- *General appearance:* Stocky appearance: Weight 169 lb, height 5 feet, 4 inches (overweight); position of comfort—two pillows propped behind lower back; facial expression pleasant.
- *Vital signs:* Temperature 98.7°F; pulse 78 beats/min; respirations 20/min; BP 145/78 mm Hg in right arm.
- *Mental status:* Alert and oriented × 3 (person, place, and time).

Inspection:
- Normal curvature noted to cervical, thoracic, and lumbar spine.
- Negative deformity noted to cervical, lumbar, and thoracic spine.

Palpation:
- Negative tenderness to spinous processes.
- Negative warmth or erythema to spinal processes.

20. What factors increase Mrs. Chu's risk for DJD?

_____

21. Aside from Mrs. Chu's history of DJD, what other factors increase her risk for back problems?

_____

22. Cluster the supporting data for the following nursing diagnoses:

a. Pain related to prolonged positions.

_____

_____

_____

b. Impaired mobility related to pain.

_____

23. Identify any additional nursing diagnoses for Mrs. Chu.

_____

_____

24. *Word jumble:* Unscramble the following words. Then unscramble the circled letters to complete the sentence: Two tests for carpal tunnel syndrome are

_____

1. (E) N O B

2. D (T) N E O N

3. M L (I) G (N) T A E

4. M (L) U B R A

5. N (P) I E S

6. A C L (N) B A E

7. R S A (L) A C

8. C I (H) R O T C A

9. (A) T G I

10. (E) S L C U M

| Name: _____ | Date: _____ |
| Course: _____ | Instructor: _____ |

Student Lab Sheet: Assessing the Musculoskeletal System

Health History

Biographical data:

Current health status: symptom analysis (PQRST):

- Pain
- Weakness
- Deformity
- ADL limitations
- Balance and coordination problems

Past health history:

- Childhood illnesses
- Hospitalizations
- Surgeries
- Serious injuries/chronic illness
- Immunizations
- Allergies (food, drugs, environmental)
- Medications (prescribed and OTC)
- Recent travel/military service

Family history:

Review of systems:

- General health status
- HEENT
- Respiratory
- Cardiovascular
- Gastrointestinal
- Genitourinary
- Neurological
- Endocrine
- Lymphatic/hematological

Psychosocial profile:

- Health practices and beliefs/self-care activities
- Typical day
- Nutritional patterns (24-hour recall)
- Activity/exercise patterns
- Recreation, pets, hobbies
- Sleep/rest patterns
- Personal habits (tobacco, alcohol, caffeine, and drugs)
- Occupational health patterns
- Socioeconomic status
- Environmental health patterns
- Roles, relationships, self-concept
- Cultural/religious influences
- Family roles/relationships
- Sexuality patterns
- Social supports
- Stress/coping

Physical Assessment

General survey:

- Vital signs
- Height
- Weight

Head-to-toe scan:

- General health status
- Integumentary
- HEENT
- Respiratory
- Cardiovascular
- Abdominal
- Genitourinary
- Neurological

Assessing the Musculoskeletal System

Area/Physical Assessment Skill	Assessment	Normal Findings Developmental/Cultural Variations	Student's Findings
Inspection	**Positions:** standing, supine, sitting		
Posture and spinal curves	Note posture in relation to environment, head position, and body alignment. Note knee position	Posture/erect head midline. Normal spinal curves noted; no kyphosis, scoliosis, or lordosis. *Normal curve of spine*	POSTURE ERECT NORMAL CURVE OF SPINE
		Knee aligned with no valgus or varus deviation	
	Draw an imaginary line from anterior superior iliac crest through knee to feet. Line should transect patella if knees are midline	Lordosis is normal in pregnancy and in toddlers	
	Inspect normal curves of spine **(cervical, thoracic, lumbar, and sacral)**		
	If you note spinal deformities, **determine whether they are structural or functional (postural)**		
	Test for kyphosis and scoliosis by having client bend from waist		
	Test for lordosis by having client flatten back against wall		

	Assessment Procedure	Normal Findings		
Gait	**Inspect gait as client walks** Note wear of shoes Note phases of gait, arm swing, cadence, base of support, stride length, and toeing **Wider base of support and shorter stride length often reflects balance problem**	Phases of gait conform; gait smooth, fluid, and rhythmic; arms swing in opposition; no toeing in or out. 2- to 4-inch base of support, 12- to 14-inch stride length. Shoes worn evenly *[handwritten]*. Toddlers, elderly, obese, and pregnant clients may have wider base of support, shorter stride length, and uneven rhythm		
Cerebellar function: Balance	Observe gait, tandem walk (heel to toe), heel and toe walk, deep knee bend. Romberg's test *[NR]* Stand close to client when performing Romberg's test. Have client stand with feet together and eyes open, then closed. Swaying is a positive Romberg's test	Coordinated, balanced gait, positive tandem walk, heel and toe walk, deep knee bend Negative Romberg's test		
Coordination	Upper extremities: finger-thumb opposition and rapid alternating movements Lower extremities: toe tapping, running heel down shin **Note dominant side (usually more coordinated)**	Coordination intact. Rapid alternating movements intact bilaterally. Positive finger-thumb opposition, toe tapping. Able to run heel down shin bilaterally		
Accuracy of movements	Assess point-to-point localization with client's eyes opened, then closed	Point-to-point localization intact bilaterally		

Assessing the Musculoskeletal System (*Continued*)

Area/Physical Assessment Skill	Assessment	Normal Findings Developmental/Cultural Variations	Student's Findings
Pronator drift	Test with eyes open, then closed; note drifting	Negative pronator drift	
Measurements	Measure arm lengths and circumferences in cm	Equal arm and leg lengths, or differences that do not exceed 1 cm	
	Arm length: measure from acromion process to tip of middle finger	Equal arm and leg circumferences, or no more than 1 cm larger on dominant side	
	Leg length: measure from anterior superior iliac crest to medial malleolus		
	To ensure accurate circumference measurements, measure at midpoint of extremity		
Palpation			
Muscle tone	Palpate muscles of upper and lower extremities in relaxed and contracted state. Note any involuntary movement, tenderness, atony, hypotony, or hypertony of muscles	Muscles at rest soft and pliable, contracted positive muscle tone, firm, no involuntary movements or tenderness	

Muscle strength	Screen strength with hand grip and foot push/leg raise Test muscle strength by noting ability to perform active ROM against resistance for face, neck, shoulders, arms, elbows, hands and wrists, hip, knees, ankles, and feet. Grade strength on a 0–5 scale Compare side to side. **Dominant side may be stronger**	All muscle groups 4 to 5/5 muscle strength. Hand grip strong and equal; foot push and leg raise against resistance strong and equal	*5*
Inspection/ Palpation	**Test muscle strength as you assess ROM of joints**	
Joints	Assess ROM, condition of skin, erythema, edema, heat, deformity, crepitus, tenderness, and stability of all joints	
TMJ	Assess as for all joints, with special attention to crepitus or clicks	Full active ROM (flex, depress, extend, elevate, side to side, protract, and retract). No tenderness, deformity, crepitus, edema, or erythema
Cervical spine (neck)	Note cervical curve	Full active ROM (flex, extend, hyperextend, rotate, lateral bend). No tenderness, crepitus, erythema, or deformity. Normal cervical curve
Scapulae	Note location, symmetry, and winging	Scapula equal over second to seventh rib, no winging
Ribs	Note condition of ribs	Ribs firm, continuous, and nontender
Shoulder	Assess as for all joints, with special attention to stability	Full active ROM (flex, extend, adduct, abduct, internal/external rotate, circumduct). Joint stable; no deformity, crepitus, or tenderness

Assessing the Musculoskeletal System (*Continued*)

Area/Physical Assessment Skill	Assessment	Normal Findings Developmental/Cultural Variations	Student's Findings
Elbows	Assess as for all joints, with special attention to nodules	Full active ROM (flex, extend, supinate, pronate). No nodules, crepitus, tenderness, or swelling	
Wrists	If indicated, assess for carpal tunnel syndrome with Tinel's test or Phalen's test	Full active ROM (flex, extend, hyperextend, radial/ulnar deviation). Joint stable, no crepitus, tenderness. Negative Tinel's and Phalen's tests	
Fingers and thumbs	Assess as for all joints, with special attention to deformities. Inspect palmar surface for shape and symmetry Heberden's nodules often on distal interphalangeal joints. Bouchard's nodules often on proximal interphalangeal joints	Full active ROM (flex, extend, hyperextend, abduct, adduct). Nontender, no deformities. Palms concave and symmetrical	
Thoracic and lumbar spine	Note thoracic and lumbar curves	Full active ROM (flex, extend, hyperextend, lateral bends, rotate)	
Hips	Assess as for all joints, with special attention to stability If indicated, do Trendelenburg test for hip dislocation If indicated, do Thomas test for hip flexure contraction	Full active ROM (flex, extend, hyperextend, internal/external rotate, abduct, adduct). Joint stable, no crepitus, nontender	

	In newborn, do Ortolani's maneuver to test for hip dislocation If sciatica present, do straight leg raise		
Knees	Assess as for all joints, with special attention to crepitus and swelling If indicated, do McMurray's and Apley's tests for foreign body, torn meniscus If indicated do drawer test, for anterior cruciate ligament and posterior cruciate ligament tears If indicated do, bulge sign or patellar tap for fluid	Full active ROM (flex, extend); knee stable; no swelling, tenderness, crepitus, or nodules	
Ankles	Assess as for all joints, with special attention to tenderness	Full active ROM (plantar flex, dorsiflex, evert, invert). No tenderness or crepitus	
Feet/toes	Assess as for all joints, with special attention to deformities, corns, bunions, hammer toes, and hallux valgus Note arch, flat feet, or high arches **Look at type of shoes client wears. They could be the cause of his or her problems**	Full active ROM (flex, extend, dorsiflex, abduct, adduct). No deformities; longitudinal arch, weight bearing on foot at midline	

Pertinent Health History Findings:

_____

_____

_____

_____

Pertinent Physical Assessment Findings:

_____

_____

_____

_____

Nursing Diagnoses (actual or potential) with Clustered Data:

_____

_____

_____

_____

Name: _____ Date: _____

Course: _____ Instructor: _____

Self-Evaluation Exercise

Musculoskeletal System	YES	NO	NEED MORE PRACTICE
1. Applies knowledge of anatomy and physiology of the musculoskeletal system in performing an assessment of the musculoskeletal system			
2. Applies growth and development principles as applicable to the musculoskeletal system			
3. Considers cultural variations as indicated when performing a musculoskeletal assessment			
4. Gathers all equipment necessary to perform a musculoskeletal assessment			
5. Obtains history specific to assessment of the musculoskeletal system			
6. Performs a physical assessment of the musculoskeletal system, including • General survey and head-to-toe scan • Inspection • Palpation			
7. Documents musculoskeletal assessment findings			
8. Identifies normal/abnormal findings			
9. Clusters pertinent subjective/objective data			
10. Identifies actual/potential health problems and states them as nursing diagnoses with supporting data			

Chapter 19

Assessing the Sensory-Neurological System

Name: _____	**Date:** _____
Course: _____	**Instructor:** _____

1. Anatomy review: Label the following structures.

- Frontal lobe

- Parietal lobe

- Temporal lobe

- Occipital lobe

- Cerebellum

- Lateral fissure

- Central fissure

- Transversal fissure

- Wernicke's area

- Broca's area

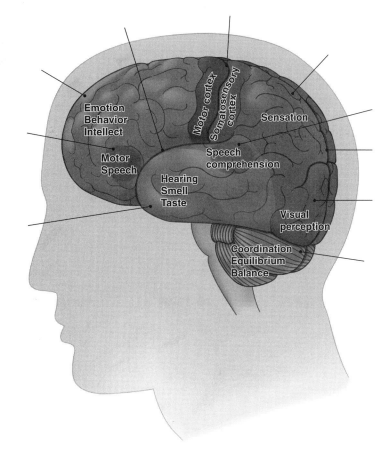

2. Match the neurological structure in the first column to the appropriate description in the second column.

   Structure

   1. Cortex
   2. Thalamus
   3. Hypothalamus
   4. Medulla
   5. Cerebellum
   6. Temporal lobe
   7. Parietal lobe
   8. Occipital lobe
   9. Frontal lobe
   10. Limbic system
   11. Reticular activating system
   12. Meninges

   Description

   a. Controls balance and coordination of movements
   b. Controls conscious process
   c. Cardiac and respiratory center
   d. Protective covering of the brain and spine
   e. Vision center
   f. Interprets cutaneous sensations
   g. Controls voluntary movement, language expression, and personality
   h. Controls hearing and language comprehension
   i. Maintains consciousness and wakefulness
   j. Regulates body temperature, appetite, and pituitary hormones
   k. Primitive drives, sexual and emotional arousal
   l. Integrates sensory stimuli

3. Diane Dubrow states that her mother-in-law Violet, age 77, seems to be getting forgetful. You begin your neurological assessment of Mrs. Dubrow by assessing her level of consciousness. Name the three areas of orientation you should test.

   PERSON, PLACE, TIME

4. If your client does not respond to verbal or tactile stimuli, what three types of painful stimuli can you use to assess response?

   STERNAL RUB, NAIL PRESSURE, ACHILLES PINCH

5. What two types of painful response should you avoid?

   NIPPLE TWIST & EYEBALL PRESSURE

6. What three types of memory should you assess to determine memory status?

   IMMEDIATE, RECENT, & REMOTE MEMORY

7. What types of memory loss are often seen in the older adult?

   RECENT & IMMEDIATE

8. If you ask your client, "What year is it?" and the client responds "2050," how would you interpret this response?

   PSYCHIATRIC PROBLEM

9. The cranial nerves are tested as part of the neurological examination. Match the cranial nerve in the first column to the appropriate test in the second column.

Cranial Nerve	**Test**
1. I: Olfactory	a. Snellen eye chart
2. II: Optic	b. Pupillary reaction
3. III: Oculomotor	c. Smell coffee
4. IV: Trochlear	d. Light touch on face
5. V: Trigeminal	e. Downward eye movement
6. VI: Abducent	f. Taste on anterior portion of tongue
7. VII: Facial	g. Test hearing
8. VIII: Acoustic	h. Taste on posterior portion of tongue
9. IX: Glossopharyngeal	i. Shoulder muscle strength
10. X: Vagus	j. Lateral eye movement
11. XI: Spinoaccessory	k. ROM of tongue
12. XII: Hypoglossal	l. Gag reflex

10. You also test DTRs. Match the DTR in the first column with the appropriate response in the second column.

Reflex	**Response**
1. Biceps	a. Knee extension
2. Triceps	b. Flexion at elbow
3. Brachioradialis	c. Plantar flexion
4. Patellar	d. Supination and flexion of wrist
5. Achilles	e. Extension at elbow

11. If you have difficulty eliciting a DTR, what two reinforcement techniques can you use to enhance the response?

_____

12. Describe the grading scale that is used to grade the DTR response.

_____

_____

13. When you assess the plantar reflex, what normal and abnormal responses might you elicit?

_____

14. What instructions should you give your client before performing a sensory examination?

_____

15. What sensation can you defer from testing if the client's pain sensation is intact? Why?

_____

_____

16. When testing deep and superficial sensations, can you assume that if sensation is intact distally, it is intact in the entire arm?

_____

17. Describe the technique for testing vibratory sensation.

_____

_____

18. Describe the technique for testing kinesthetic sensation.

_____

_____

19. Match the discriminatory sensation in the first column with the appropriate response in the second column.

Sensation	**Response**
1. Graphesthesia	a. Able to identify site that was stimulated
2. Stereognosis	b. Able to identify simultaneous stimuli on opposite sides of body
3. Two-point discrimination	c. Able to identify written number/letter on palm
4. Extinction	d. Able to identify two simultaneous stimuli on skin, closing in until indiscernible
5. Point localization	e. Able to identify object through touch

20. Although your assessment focuses on the sensory/neurological system, all systems are related. What assessment findings (subjective or objective) show the relationship between the sensory/neurological system and other systems?

_____

_____

_____

<table>
<tr><td>Name: _____</td><td>Date: _____</td></tr>
<tr><td>Course: _____</td><td>Instructor: _____</td></tr>
</table>

PULSE PRESSURE
DISTOLYIC - SYSTOLIC.

Abnormal Case Study: Leon Webster

Leon Webster is a 21-year-old, black college senior. On Friday night, he and several friends went to a local club to celebrate the basketball team's winning season. While driving home, his car hit a tree. He is brought to the ED 30 minutes later by ambulance. Leon is alert and oriented, complaining of a headache and neck pain. He has a 3-inch laceration on his forehead where his head hit the rearview mirror. He was not wearing a seat belt. He was treated in the ED and discharged home with instructions and referral for follow-up.

Three hours later, the client's mother brings him back to the ED, saying, "Leon says his head really hurts." She states that he cannot keep any food down, that he vomited two times, and that she had a hard time keeping him awake on the ride to the hospital. Because there has been a drastic change in Leon's condition, a focused neurological assessment is indicated.

Health History

- History of head trauma 5 hours earlier.
- No medication.
- Had been drinking alcohol before accident.
- No history or other neurological or medical problems.
- No known drug allergies.
- Worsening headache and sleepy.

Physical Assessment

- *General appearance:* Well-groomed; speech clear, but slow; slumped posture; guarding head and neck; sleepy, yet grimacing in pain.
- *Vital signs:* Temperature 98°F; pulse 60 beats/min, regular; respirations 20/min; BP 150/60 mm Hg; pulse oximetry 98% room air.
- *Integumentary:* Two-inch sutured laceration on forehead; otherwise negative.

- *HEENT:* Facial features symmetrical; pupils 5 mm equal but sluggish reaction.
- *Respiratory:* Lungs clear.
- *Cardiovascular:* Heart sounds 60 beats/min and regular, no extra sounds.
- *Abdomen:* Soft, nontender, positive bowel sounds.
- *Musculoskeletal:* +4/5 strength of upper and lower extremities; decreased ROM of neck.
- *Level of consciousness:* Awake, alert, and oriented × 3 but lethargic, falling asleep, Glasgow Coma Scale 14.
- *Communication:* Intact but slow.
- *Memory:* Immediate, remote intact, but doesn't remember events of accident.
- *Cognitive functions:* Too lethargic to test.
- CN I through XII intact; DTR +2, positive plantar.

(#1st AROUSAL)

21. What may account for the change in Leon's assessment findings?

INTERCRANIAL PRESSURE INCREASE (NAUSEA, BP↑, CONCIOUSNESS, HEAD ACHE)

22. What is one of the earliest signs of a change in neurological status?

SPECH IMPAIRMENT, VOMITING, PAIN, LETHARGIN

23. Which of Leon's findings would alert you to a change in intracranial pressure?

   NAUSEA, BP↑, CONCIOUSNESS, AROUSAL, HEADACHE

24. Cluster the supporting data for the following nursing diagnoses:

   a. Ineffective cerebral tissue perfusion related to response to injury.

   PRESSURE SO GREAT TISSUES DONT HAVE NEEDED OXYGEN.
   SLURRED SPEACH, HEADACHE, DIALATED PUPILS.

   b. Pain related to head and neck trauma.

   GRIMACING IN PAIN
   NECK & HEAD PAIN

25. Identify any additional nursing diagnoses for Leon.

26. *Word jumble:* Unscramble the following words. Then unscramble the circled letters to complete the sentence: The universal tool used to assess level of consciousness is

   1. N B (A) I R

   2. X (C) T R O E

   3. (L) H A S M U T

   4. Y P A (S) N E S

   5. (E) F R A E T N F

   6. (S) R N O U N E

   7. M L B R C E (L) U E E

   8. E L U D M L (A)

   9. E K I (W) R E N C

   10. S A C R B (O) R (A) E A

   11. R Y A (G) R T E T A M

   12. E B M U R E (C)

   13. N (G) I N S E M E

   14. C P T I C (O) I A L   B O L E

Name: _____ Date: _____

Course: _____ Instructor: _____

Student Lab: Assessing the Sensory-Neurological System

Health History

Biographical data:

Current health status: symptom analysis (PQRST):

- Headaches
- Dizziness
- Seizures
- Loss of consciousness
- Change in sensation
- Change in mobility
- Dysphagia (difficulty swallowing)
- Dysphasia (difficulty speaking)

Past health history:

- Childhood illnesses
- Hospitalizations
- Surgeries
- Serious injuries/chronic illness
- Immunizations
- Allergies (food, drugs, environmental)
- Medications (prescribed and OTC)
- Recent travel/military service

Family history:

Review of systems:

- General health status
- HEENT
- Respiratory
- Cardiovascular
- Gastrointestinal
- Genitourinary
- Musculoskeletal
- Endocrine

- Lymphatic/hematological

Psychosocial profile:

- Health practices and beliefs/self-care activities
- Typical day
- Nutritional patterns (24-hour recall)
- Activity/exercise patterns
- Recreation, pets, hobbies
- Sleep/rest patterns
- Personal habits (tobacco, alcohol, caffeine, and drugs)
- Occupational health patterns
- Socioeconomic status
- Environmental health patterns
- Roles, relationships, self-concept
- Cultural/religious influences
- Family roles/relationships
- Sexuality patterns
- Social supports
- Stress/coping

General survey:

- Vital signs
- Height
- Weight

Head-to-toe scan:

- General health status
- Integumentary
- HEENT
- Respiratory
- Cardiovascular
- Abdominal
- Genitourinary
- Musculoskeletal

Assessing the Sensory-Neurological System

Area/Physical Assessment Skill	Assessment	Normal Findings Developmental/Cultural Variations	Student's Findings
	Position: sitting		
Cerebral function	**Consider client's age, educational and cultural background**		
Behavior	Note facial expression, posture, affect, and grooming	Well-groomed, erect posture, pleasant facial expression, appropriate affect Normal findings vary depending on situation	
Level of consciousness	Test orientation to time, place, and person Disorientation to time/place usually occurs before disorientation to person	Awake alert and oriented × 3 (time, place, and person) Older clients may be disoriented to time, but note if they reorient easily	
Memory	Test immediate, recent, and remote memory Immediate: Ask client to repeat a series of numbers Recent: Name three objects and ask client to recall them later in exam Remote: Ask client his or her birth date and date of major historical event **If asking for personal data, such as birth date, be sure you can validate information**	Immediate, recent, and remote memory intact	

Mathematical/ calculative ability	Have client perform simple mathematical problem, such as 4 + 5, serial 7s or 4s, subtracting from 100	Calculative skills intact
General knowledge	Assess vocabulary and general knowledge Ask how many days in a week or months in a year or for definition of familiar words. **Begin with easy words and proceed to more difficult ones (e.g., apple, earthquake, chastise)**	Vocabulary appropriate and general knowledge intact
Thought process	Note attention span, logic of speech, ability to stay focused, appropriateness of responses	Thought process clear, responds appropriately, speech coherent and logical
Abstract thinking	Give client a proverb to interpret Have client identify similarities, such as apples and oranges	Abstract thinking intact
Judgment	Assess client's response to hypothetical situations	Judgment intact
Communication	Note speech and language, enunciation, fluency. Note any dysarthria (difficulty with articulation), dysphasia (difficulty with speech), dysphonia (difficulty/change in voice quality), neologisms (meaningless words), circumlocution (inability to name objects verbally) Test spontaneous speech by having client describe a picture	Speech clear, fluent; no dysarthria, dysphasia, dysphonia, neologisms, or circumlocution Communication skills intact: spontaneous speech, automatic speech, motor speech, sound recognition, auditory-verbal comprehension, visual recognition, visual-verbal comprehension, writing and copying figures

Assessing the Sensory-Neurological System (*Continued*)

Area/Physical Assessment Skill	Assessment	Normal Findings Developmental/Cultural Variations	Student's Findings
	Test motor speech by having client say, "doe, ray, me, fa, so, la, te, doe"		
	Test automatic speech by having client recite days of week		
	Test sound recognition by having client identify familiar sounds		
	Test auditory-verbal comprehension by noting client's ability to follow directions		
	Test visual recognition by having client identify objects by sight		
	Test visual-verbal comprehension by having client read a sentence and explain meaning		
	Test writing by having client write name and address		
	Test copying figures by having client copy a circle, x, square, triangle, and star		
	Start with simple tasks and work to more complex ones		
Cranial nerves	**Compare side to side**		
	Have client close eyes when testing sensory nerves		

CN I—olfactory	Check patency of nostrils. Test each separately. Note anosmia Have client identify a distinct odor (coffee, vanilla)	CN I intact Sense of smell intact
CN II—optic	Test visual acuity, visual fields, retinal structures	CN II intact Visual acuity intact
CN III—oculomotor CN IV—trochlear CN VI—abducent	Test EOM with 6 cardinal fields, check pupillary reaction to light and accommodation If indicated, test oculocephalic reflex ***Alert: Never test oculocephalic reflex (doll's eyes) on a client with suspected neck injury***	CN III, IV, VI intact Extraocular muscles intact OU, PERRLA direct and consensual
CN V—trigeminal	Test jaw (mastication) muscle strength by having client bite down on tongue blade Test sensations on face (forehead, cheeks, chin) Test corneal reflex	CN V intact Jaw muscle strength +5, facial sensations intact, positive corneal reflex
CN VII—facial	Test motor function of facial muscles by having client make faces, smile, frown, and whistle Test taste (sweet, sour, salty) on anterior portion of tongue	CN VII intact Facial movements symmetrical Taste on anterior tongue intact
CN VIII—acoustic nerve	Test hearing, balance If indicated, do cold caloric test (oculovestibular reflex) and look for nystagmus (normal response)	CN VIII intact Hearing and balance intact

Assessing the Sensory-Neurological System (*Continued*)

Area/Physical Assessment Skill	Assessment	Normal Findings Developmental/Cultural Variations	Student's Findings
CN IX and X—glossopharyngeal and vagus nerves	Note quality of voice, ability to swallow and cough. Test gag reflex. Look for symmetrical rise of the uvula Assess taste on posterior third of tongue	CN IX and X intact Strong, clear voice, symmetrical rise of uvula, able to swallow and cough Positive gag reflex Taste on posterior tongue intact	
CN XI—spinal accessory nerve	Test muscle strength of neck and shoulders	CN XI intact +5 muscle strength of neck and shoulders	
CN XII—hypoglossal nerve	Test mobility and strength of tongue. Note ability to say "d, l, n, t" Note tongue position, atrophy, or fasciculation	CN XII intact Full ROM of tongue, midline, no atrophy or fasciculation	
Sensory function	**Have client close eyes. Compare side to side**		
Light touch, pain, and temperature	Test light touch, pain, and temperature on various areas of body **If touch sensation intact distally, do not assume it is intact proximally** **If pain sensation intact, no need to test temperature** **Avoid using pin because it could break skin. Use sharp and dull sides of toothpick to test pain**	Light touch, pain, and temperature intact upper and lower extremities	

Deep sensation: vibratory and kinesthetic (position sense) sensations	Place vibrating tuning fork on bony joint, great toe, and distal interphalangeal joint Move finger and toe up and down, and have client identify direction of movement **If intact distally, intact proximally**	Vibratory and kinesthetic sensations intact upper and lower extremities
Discriminatory sensations: Stereognosis Graphesthesia Two-point discrimination Point localization Extinction	Stereognosis: Have client identify familiar object (key, paper clip) by touch Graphesthesia: Draw number or letter in palm of hand and have client identify Two-point discrimination: Note ability to differentiate being touched at one or two points simultaneously. **Ability to discriminate depends on area tested. Fingertips are most discriminatory** Point localization: Note ability to identify a point touched Extinction: Note ability to identify two corresponding areas touched simultaneously	Stereognosis, graphesthesia, two-point discrimination < 5 mm on fingertips, point localization and extinction intact
DTRs	**Grade DTRs on 0–4 scale** **If difficulty eliciting reflex, use reinforcement techniques: clenching teeth, interlocking hands** **Use percussion hammer**	

KNOW THESE

Assessing the Sensory-Neurological System (*Continued*)

Area/Physical Assessment Skill	Assessment	Normal Findings Developmental/Cultural Variations	Student's Findings
Biceps (C5, C6)	Place your thumb on biceps tendon and strike Response: Flexion at elbow	+2/4	
Triceps (C7, C8)	Strike triceps tendon 1 to 2 inches above elbow Response: Extension at elbow	+2/4	
Brachioradialis (C5, C6)	Strike brachioradialis tendon 3 to 5 cm above wrist Response: Flexion at elbow and supination of hand	+2/4	
Patellar (L2, L3, L4)	Strike patellar tendon below patella Response: Extension of the knees	+2/4	
Achilles (S1, S2)	Strike Achilles tendon about 2 inches above heel Response: Plantar flexion of the foot	+2/4	
Superficial reflexes	**Grade as positive or negative**		
Plantar (L4 to S2)	Stroke sole of foot from heel laterally across ball of foot to great toe Response: Flexion of toes **Babinski response: Dorsiflexion of great toe and fanning of toes**	Positive plantar reflex Babinski normal in infants	

Abdominal (T8, T9, T10)	Stroke each quadrant of abdomen toward umbilicus Response: Umbilicus moves toward stimulus	Positive abdominal reflex May be absent in obese or pregnant clients
Anal (S3, S4, S5)	Scratch side of anus Response: Puckering of anus	Positive anal reflex
Cremasteric (L1, L2)	Stroke inner aspect of male's thigh Response: Elevation of testes	Positive cremasteric reflex
Bulbocavernous (S3, S4)	Gently apply pressure over bulbocavernous muscle and gently pinch foreskin or glans Response: Contraction of bulbocavernous muscle	Positive bulbocavernous reflex

Pertinent Health History Findings:

_____

_____

_____

_____

Pertinent Physical Assessment Findings:

_____

_____

_____

_____

Nursing Diagnoses (actual or potential) with Clustered Data:

_____

_____

_____

_____

Name: _____	Date: _____
Course: _____	Instructor: _____

Self-Evaluation Exercise

Sensory-Neurological System	YES	NO	NEED MORE PRACTICE
1. Applies knowledge of anatomy and physiology of the sensory-neurological system in performing an assessment of the sensory-neurological system			
2. Applies growth and development principles as applicable to the sensory-neurological system			
3. Considers cultural variations as indicated when performing a sensory-neurological assessment			
4. Gathers all equipment necessary to perform a sensory-neurological assessment			
5. Obtains history specific to assessment of the sensory-neurological system			
6. Perform a physical assessment of the sensory-neurological system, including • General survey and head-to-toe scan • Inspection • Palpation • Reflexes			
7. Documents sensory-neurological assessment findings			
8. Identifies normal/abnormal findings.			
9. Clusters pertinent subjective/objective data.			
10. Identifies actual/potential health problems and states them as nursing diagnoses with supporting data.			

Chapter 20
Putting It All Together

Sample Assessment Form

Health History
Biographical data:

Name: _____

Address: _____

Phone number: _____

Contact person (relationship to client): _____

Age: _____   Marital status: _____

Birth date: _____   Number of dependents: _____

Birthplace: _____   Educational level: _____

Gender: _____   Occupation: _____

Ethnicity/nationality: _____   Advance directive: _____

Social Security number: _____   Health insurance: _____

Referral (primary care physician/practitioner): _____

Source of history/reliability: _____

Reason for seeking health care:

_____

_____

Past health history:

Childhood illnesses: _____

Hospitalizations: _____

Surgeries: _____

Serious injuries/chronic illnesses: _____

Immunizations: _____

Allergies (food, drugs, environmental): _____

Medications (prescribed/OTC): _____

Recent travel/military service: _____

Family History:

_____

_____

Review of systems:

General health status: _____

Integumentary: _____

Skin _____

Hair _____

Nails _____

HEENT: _____

Head and neck: _____

Eyes: _____

Ears: _____

Nose and sinuses: _____

Mouth and throat: _____

Respiratory: _____

Cardiovascular: _____

Breasts: _____

Gastrointestinal: _____

Genitourinary: _____

Female/male reproductive: _____

Musculoskeletal: _____

Neurological: _____

Endocrine: _____

Immune/hematological: _____

Developmental:

_____

_____

Psychosocial profile:

Health practices and beliefs/self-care activities: _____

Typical day: _____

Nutritional patterns (24-hour recall): _____

Activity/exercise patterns: _____

Recreation, pets, hobbies: _____

Sleep/rest patterns: _____

Personal habits (tobacco, alcohol, caffeine, and drugs): _____

Occupational health patterns: _____

Socioeconomic status: _____

Environmental health patterns: _____

Roles, relationships, self-concept: _____

Cultural/religious influences: _____

Family roles/relationships: _____

Sexuality patterns: _____

Social supports: _____

Stress/coping patterns: _____

Summary of Pertinent Health History Findings:

_____

_____

Physical Assessment

General appearance:

Vital signs: Temperature _____; pulse _____; respirations _____; BP (left/right) _____

Height: _____

Weight: _____

Integumentary: _____

HEENT: _____

Head and neck: _____

Eyes: _____

Ears: _____

Nose and sinuses: _____

Mouth and throat: _____

Respiratory: _____

Cardiovascular: _____

Breasts: _____

Abdomen: _____

Female/male reproductive: _____

Musculoskeletal: _____

Neurological: _____

Endocrine: _____

Lymphatic/hematological: _____

Summary of Pertinent Physical Assessment Findings:

_____

_____

Name: _____	*Date:* _____
Course: _____	*Instructor:* _____

Assessment Form "Guide at a Glance"

Health History

Biographical data:

Name: _____

Address: _____

Phone number: _____

Contact person (relationship to client): _____

Age: _____ Marital status: _____

Birth date: _____ Number of dependents: _____

Birthplace: _____ Educational level: _____

Gender: _____ Occupation: _____

Ethnicity/nationality: _____ Advance directive: _____

Social security number: _____ Health insurance: _____

Referral (primary care physician/practitioner): _____

Source of history/reliability: _____

Reason for seeking health care:

Primary level: Include usual state of health, any major health problems, usual patterns of health care, and health concerns.

Secondary and tertiary levels: Identify chief complaint and do symptom analysis (PQRST).

Past Health History

Childhood illnesses: Ask about mumps, chickenpox, rubella, ear infections, streptococcal infections or sore throats, scarlet fever, pertussis, and asthma.

Hospitalizations: Include name of hospital, reason for hospitalization, physician name, dates, and length of stay.

Surgeries: Include surgical procedures, physician name, and hospital.

Serious injuries: Include head injuries with loss of consciousness, fractures, motor vehicle accidents, burns, and lacerations.

Chronic illnesses: Include heart disease, HTN, diabetes, cancer, and seizures.

Immunizations: Age dependent; include measles, mumps, rubella, tetanus, diphtheria, pertussis, chickenpox, hepatitis B, polio, *Haemophilus influenzae* B (HIB), pneumococcal vaccine, influenza, meningitis, tuberculosis testing.

Allergies: Include food, drug, and environmental allergens and whether client ever had penicillin. If positive for allergy, state type of reaction.

Medications: Include prescribed and OTC, including vitamin and herbal supplements. Assess client's understanding of medications.

Recent travel/military service: Include travel within past year and recent and past military service.

Family History

Include client, spouse, children, parents, siblings, aunts, uncles, and grandparents. List family members or draw a genogram.

Review of Systems

General health status: Ask about fatigue, exercise intolerance, unexplained fever, night sweats, weakness, difficulty with ADL, and number of colds and illnesses per year.

Integumentary:

Skin: Ask about skin diseases, itching, rashes, scars, sores, ulcers, warts, moles, changes in skin lesions, and skin reactions to hot and cold.

Hair: Ask about changes in hair texture, baldness, unusual patterns, and hair care (e.g., shampoo, coloring, permanents).

Nails: Ask about changes in nails, color, texture, splitting, cracking, and nail care (e.g., use of polish or acrylic nails).

HEENT:

Head and neck: Ask about headaches, lumps, scars, recent head trauma, injury or surgery, history of concussion, loss of consciousness, dizzy spells, fainting, stiff neck, pain with head movement, swollen glands, and nodes or masses.

Eyes: Ask about use of corrective lenses (glasses or contact lenses), visual deficits, last eye examination, last glaucoma check, eye injury, itching, tearing, drainage, pain, floaters, halos, loss of vision of parts of fields, blurred vision, double vision, colored lights, flashing lights, light sensitivity, twitching, cataracts, glaucoma, eye surgery, retinal detachment, strabismus, and amblyopia.

Ears: Ask about last hearing test, difficulty hearing, sensitivity to sounds, ear pain, drainage, vertigo, ear infections, ringing, fullness, wax problems, use of hearing aids, and ear care habits.

Nose and sinuses: Ask about nosebleeds, broken nose, deviated septum, snoring, postnasal drip, runny nose, sneezing, allergies, use of recreational drugs, difficulty breathing through nose, problem with ability to smell, pain over sinuses, sinus infections.

Mouth and throat: Ask about sore throats, streptococcal infections, mouth sores, oral herpes, bleeding gums, hoarseness, changes in quality of voice, difficulty chewing or swallowing, changes in sense of taste, dentures and bridges, dental health and hygiene patterns, dental surgery, and date of last dental examination.

Respiratory: Ask about breathing problems, cough, sputum (color and amount), shortness of breath with activity, noisy respirations, pneumonia, tuberculosis, bronchitis, last chest x-ray, PPD and results, and history of smoking.

Cardiovascular: Ask about chest pain, palpitations, murmurs, skipped beats, HTN, awakening at night, shortness of breath, dizzy spells, cold or numb hands and feet, color changes in hands and feet, swelling of extremities, hair loss on legs, sores that do not heal, and ECGs and results.

Breasts: Ask about breast masses, lumps, pain, discharge, swelling, changes in breasts or nipples, cystic breast disease, breast cancer, breast surgery, reduction/enhancement, BSE (when and how), date of last clinical breast examination, and mammograms and results.

Gastrointestinal: Ask about appetite and changes, indigestion, heartburn, gastroesophageal reflux disease, nausea, vomiting, vomiting blood, liver or gallbladder disease, jaundice, abdominal swelling, bowel patterns and changes, color and consistency of stools, diarrhea, constipation, hemorrhoids, weight changes, use of laxatives, antacids, date and results of last fecal occult blood test, and colonoscopies and results.

Genitourinary: Ask about pain on urination, burning, frequency, urgency, dribbling, incontinence, hesitancy, changes in urine stream, color of urine, history of urinary tract infections, kidney infections, kidney disease, kidney stones, and frequent nighttime urination.

Female/male reproductive: *Female*: Ask about menarche, description of cycle, LMP, painful menses, excessive bleeding, irregular menses, bleeding between periods, last Pap test and results, satisfaction with sexual performance, painful intercourse, use of contraceptives, STDs, knowledge of STD prevention, safe sex practices, infertility problems, pregnancies, live births, miscarriages, and abortions. *Male*: Ask about lesions, discharge, pain on urination, painful intercourse, prostate or scrotal problems, history of STDs, knowledge of STD prevention, safe sex practices, infertility problems, impotence or sterility, satisfaction with sexual performance, frequency and technique for TSE, and last prostate examination and results.

Musculoskeletal: Ask about fractures, sprains, muscle cramps, pain, weakness, joint swelling, redness, limited ROM, joint deformity, noise with movement, spinal deformities, low back pain, loss of height, osteoporosis, DJD, rheumatoid arthritis, use of calcium supplements, ability to do ADL, and bone density scan and results.

Neurological: Ask about loss of consciousness; fainting; seizures; head injury; changes in cognition; memory; hallucinations; disorientation; speech problems; sensory deficits such as numbness, tingling, and loss of sensation; motor problems; problems with gait, balance, and coordination; and ability to do ADL.

Endocrine: Ask about thyroid disease; diabetes; changes in weight, thirst, hunger, or urination; heat and cold intolerance; goiter; weakness; hormone therapy; and changes in skin and hair.

Lymphatic/hemotological: Ask about bleeding disorders, recurrent infections, cancers, HIV, fatigue, blood transfusions, bruising, allergies, and unexplained swollen nodes.

Developmental: Identify current developmental level and prior developmental problems.

Psychosocial Profile

Health practices and beliefs/self-care activities: Ask about perceived health, what client does to stay healthy, yearly physical examinations, self- examinations.

Typical day: Ask about usual day from time client awakens until bedtime.

Nutritional patterns: Do a 24-hour recall and compare with food groups. Use weekday diet.

Activity/exercise patterns: Ask about types and amounts of exercise and use of protective equipment.

Recreation, pets, hobbies: Identify health risk factors.

Sleep/rest patterns: Ask about number of hours of sleep per night, whether sleep is restful, naps, and use of sleep aids.

Personal habits (tobacco, alcohol, caffeine, and drugs): Ask about type, amount, and years used.

Occupational health patterns: Identify health risks or exposure to toxic substances.

Socioeconomic status: Ask about health insurance.

Environmental health patterns: Identify environment as urban/rural; ask about safety of home and neighborhood, type of home, heating and plumbing, and smoke detectors.

Roles, relationships, self-concept: Ask about roles/relationships and how client sees self.

Cultural/religious influences: Identify cultural and religious influences on health.

Family roles/relationships: Identify client's role in family and number of dependents in family.

Sexuality patterns: Identify sexual patterns, preferences, and safe sex practices.

Social supports: Identify supports, family, friends, coworkers, and community agencies.

Stress/coping patterns: Identify amount of stress and coping mechanisms.

Physical Assessment

Head-to-Toe Physical Assessment: General Survey

General appearance: Include age, general appearance, grooming, hygiene, odors, nutritional status, level of consciousness, speech, affect, gait, posture, movements, gross deformities, and signs of distress.

Vital signs: Temperature _____; pulse _____; respirations _____; BP (left/right) _____ Height: _____ Weight: _____

Integumentary: Inspect color and lesions and palpate temperature, turgor, and texture throughout examination.

HEENT

Head: Inspect size, shape and symmetry, position, hair distribution, and lesions; palpate scalp mobility, tenderness, and hair texture.

Face: Inspect symmetry of nasolabial folds and palpebral fissures; palpate temporal arteries and TMJ; test ROM; and test facial sensations (CN V), facial expressions, and ability to smile and frown (CN VII).

Eyes: Test visual acuity near/far with Snellen chart (CN II), color vision, peripheral vision by confrontation, extraocular movement in six cardinal fields (CN III, IV, and VI), and corneal light reflex; perform cover-uncover test; test corneal blink reflex; inspect external structures (general appearance of eyes, lids, sclera, conjunctiva, cornea, lens, and anterior chamber of the iris; palpate lacrimal glands and ducts; test pupils; and perform funduscopic examination of disk, arteries and veins, fundus, and macula.

Ears: Inspect/palpate external ear; check angle of attachment; perform Weber, Rinne, and whisper tests (CN VIII); and perform otoscopic examination of canal and tympanic membrane.

Nose and sinuses: Palpate sinuses for tenderness and nasal patency; test sense of smell (CN I); and inspect nasal mucosa, septum, and turbinates.

Mouth: Inspect/palpate lips, oral mucosa, teeth, and gingiva; inspect tongue; test taste on anterior/posterior tongue (CN VII, IX); test mobility of tongue (CN XII); test gag/swallow reflex (CN IX, X); and palpate parotid and submandibular glands.

Neck: Inspect, palpate, and auscultate thyroid gland; palpate and auscultate carotids; measure jugular venous pressure; palpate nodes and tracheal position; note ROM of neck; and test neck muscle strength (CN XI).

Posterior thorax/lungs: Palpate excursion and fremitus, percuss lungs and diaphragmatic excursion, and auscultate breath sounds.

Posterior thorax/spine: Inspect normal spinal curves; test for scoliosis, kyphosis, and lordosis; check ROM of spine; palpate paravertebral muscles for tenderness; fist/blunt percuss costovertebral angle tenderness.

Anterior thorax/breast: Inspect and palpate breast and lymph nodes with client in various positions.

Anterior thorax/lungs: Inspect antero-posterior:lateral ratio, palpate excursion and fremitus, percuss chest, and auscultate breath sounds.

Anterior thorax/heart: Inspect and palpate precordium for pulsations, note PMI, and auscultate heart sounds.

Upper extremities: Palpate brachial, radial, and ulnar pulses; perform Allen's test if indicated; perform Tinel's or Phalen's test for carpal tunnel syndrome if indicated; check color, temperature, capillary refill, deformities, and clubbing of hands and nails; inspect joints for deformities; test hand grip; check ROM and strength; measure arm length and circumferences; test pronator drift; test coordination with rapid alternating movements and finger-thumb opposition; test accuracy of movements with point-to-point localization; test superficial and deep sensations; and test DTR of upper extremities.

Abdomen: Inspect size, shape, symmetry, and movements (respirations, pulsations, and peristalsis); test for hernias; auscultate bowel and vascular sounds; percuss abdomen and organs; if ascites suspected, percuss for shifting dullness; and palpate abdominal organs (liver, kidneys and spleen), aorta, inguinal lymph nodes, and femoral arteries.

Lower extremities: Inspect color, hair distribution, and varicose veins; perform Trendelenburg test or manual compression test to check venous circulation, if indicated; palpate pedal pulses and temperature; inspect condition of feet and toenails and note lesions and deformities; test ROM of lower extremities; measure leg lengths and circumferences; perform straight leg test if indicated; perform patellar tap or bulge sign if fluid suspected; check for drawer sign if torn anterior cruciate ligament or posterior cruciate ligament suspected; perform Apley's or McMurray's test if meniscus tear suspected; test muscle strength and superficial and deep sensations; inspect gait, toe and heel walking, tandem walk, and deep knee bend; perform Romberg's test; have client toe tap and run heel down shin; and test Achilles, patellar DTR, and plantar reflexes.

Female genitalia/rectum: Inspect and palpate external and internal genitalia, obtain specimens as indicated, inspect and palpate rectum for masses, and test stool for occult blood.

Male genitalia/rectum: Inspect and palpate male genitalia, inspect and palpate rectum for masses, and test stool for occult blood.

Using the Four Techniques of Physical Assessment by System

Integumentary:

Skin:

Inspect: Color, lesions (note location, distribution, configuration, and morphology), and vascular lesions.

Palpate: Moisture, temperature, texture, elasticity (turgor), and masses.

Hair:

Inspect: Color and distribution.

Palpate: Texture.

Nails:

Inspect: Color, angle of attachment, and markings.

Palpate: Texture and capillary refill.

HEENT:

Head and face:

Inspect: Size, shape, symmetry, nasolabial folds, palpebral fissures, edema, pigmentation, lesions, tics, and grimacing.

Palpate: Skull and mobility of scalp.

Neck:

Inspect: Three positions (neutral, hyperextended, and as client swallows), anterior and posterior triangles, and trachea.

Palpate: Trachea, lymph nodes, and thyroid.

Eyes:

Test visual acuity: Near/far vision, peripheral vision, color vision, position and alignment of extraocular muscles, corneal light reflex, six cardinal fields, and cover-uncover test.

Inspect: General appearance, lashes, lids, conjunctiva, sclera, cornea, anterior chamber, iris, and pupils.

Palpate: Lacrimal glands and ducts.

Funduscopic: Vessels, disk, retina, and macula.

Ears:

Test hearing: Whispered voice sounds, Weber test, and Rinne test.

Inspect: Angle of attachment, position and drainage, and shape and symmetry.

Palpate: Consistency, nodules, tragus, mastoid, and pull helix forward.

Otoscopic examination: External ear canal: color, patency, drainage; tympanic membrane: color, drainage, landmarks, intactness, and mobility of drum.

Nose:

Inspect: Position, drainage, septal deviation, nasal mucosa, and turbinates.

Palpate: Nasal patency and tenderness.

Sinuses:

Inspect: Edema.

Palpate: Tenderness.

Percuss: Tenderness.

Transilluminate: fluid.

Mouth and throat:

Inspect: Note odor of breath.

Lips: Color, lesions, hydration. *Teeth:* Number, condition, color, and occlusion. *Gingivae:* Color, bleeding, and retraction or hypertrophy. *Oral mucosa:* Color, lesions. *Tongue:* Color, hydration, mobility, Stensen's and Wharton's ducts, patency, and inflammation. *Tonsils:* Color, size, and exudates. *Palates:* Color and intactness. *Uvula:* Position and symmetry. *Pharynx:* Color and exudates.

Palpate: Parotid, submandibular, and sublingual glands.

Respiratory:

Inspect: Respirations, rate, rhythm, size, shape, symmetry, anteroposterior:lateral ratio, excursion, muscles of breathing, and condition of skin.

Palpate: Chest for tenderness, crepitus, tactile fremitus, and excursion.

Percuss: Chest for resonance and diaphragmatic excursion.

Auscultate: Breath sounds (vesicular, bronchovesicular, and bronchial), abnormal sounds, adventitious sounds, and abnormal voice sounds.

Cardiovascular:

Inspect: Neck vein distention, pulsations on neck and precordium, measure jugular venous pressure.

Palpate: Pulses: rate, rhythm, equality, amplitude, contour and elasticity, and thrills; precordial sites for pulsations, thrills, lifts, and heaves.

Percuss: Cardiac borders.

Auscultate: Normal heart sounds (intensity, pitch, timing in cardiac cycle, location, and splits), extra sounds OS, ejection click, S_3, S_4, murmurs and rubs, bruits, and venous hums.

Breasts:

Inspect: Positions (sitting hands at side, hands pressed on hips, hands over head, leaning forward, and supine with small pillow under shoulder of breast being examined), size, shape, symmetry, color, condition of skin, lesions, venous pattern, dimpling, retraction, masses, nipple position, inverted/everted, discharge, and axilla (color, rashes, and masses).

Palpate: Three levels (light, medium, and deep pressure), consistency, masses, tenderness, nipples for discharge, and lymph node enlargement.

Abdomen:

Inspect: Size, shape, symmetry, movements (respiratory, pulsations, and peristalsis), hernias, skin condition, venous pattern lesions, and umbilicus color and position (inverted or everted).

Auscultate: Bowel sounds, vascular sounds and rubs; scratch test.

Palpate: Light: surface characteristics; deep: abdominal organs (liver, spleen, and kidneys), rebound tenderness, rigidity, and aortic pulsation and size.

Percuss: Abdomen, liver, spleen, and kidneys for costovertebral angle tenderness; bladder for distention; and shifting dullness if ascites.

Female/Male Reproductive:

Female:

Inspect: External genitalia, vaginal mucosa, and cervix.

Palpate: Vaginal wall, cervix, uterus, adnexa, and rectum.

Obtain: Specimens as indicated.

Male:

Inspect: External genitalia, penis and scrotum, and inguinal area.

Palpate: Penis, scrotum and testes, inguinal hernias, inguinal nodes, rectum, and prostate.

Obtain: Specimens as indicated.

Musculoskeletal:

Inspect: Posture, gait, spinal curves (cervical, thoacic, lumbar, and sacral), joints (condition of skin, deformities, stability, crepitus, erythema, and ROM), cerebellar function (balance, coordination, and accuracy of movements), and limb measurements.

Palpate: Muscle tone, strength, joint deformities, tenderness, and heat.

Percuss: Patella for fluid.

Neurological:

Test:

Cerebral function: Level of consciousness, memory, communication, mental status, thought process, affect, judgment, vocabulary, and calculation.

Cranial nerves: CN I through XII.

Sensory: Superficial: light touch, pain, temperature; deep: vibratory, kinesthetic, graphesthesia, stereognosis, two-point discrimination, extinction, and point localization.

DTRs: Biceps, triceps, brachioradialis, patellar, and Achilles (grade 0–4)

Superficial reflexes: Plantar, abdominal, cremasteric, and bulbocavernosus.

Summary of Pertinent Physical Assessment Findings

Name: _____   Date: _____

Course: _____   Instructor: _____

Abnormal Case Study: Harry Holsvick

Harry Holsvick is a 32-year-old, white, male construction worker with two children. You are seeing him in the clinic for a health risk assessment.

Health History

Biographical data

- Construction worker.
- Married with two children (ages 2 and 5).
- Roman Catholic.

Current health status

- No current health problems.
- No known drug, environmental, or food allergies.
- Concerned about his father's recent heart attack and his own future heath risks.
- Seeks a health risk screening.
- No current prescription medications. Occasionally uses OTC medications for colds or headaches and takes ibuprofen for work-related aches and pains about 2 days per week.

Past health history

- No history of medical problems.
- Had chickenpox as a child.
- Leg laceration last year from falling piece of construction equipment. Healed with no complications.
- Had all childhood immunizations. Most recent tetanus last year after leg injury. Cannot remember if he had a PPD.
- No surgeries. Was hospitalized once as a teenager after a football injury when he lost consciousness for several minutes. Has been to the ED twice in past 5 years for injuries suffered on the job.

Family history

- Mother, age 64, alive and well.
- Father, age 67, HTN and recent myocardial infarction.
- Sisters, ages 27 and 34, alive and well.
- Maternal grandmother, age 85, HTN.
- Maternal grandfather, died of myocardial infarction at age 81.
- Maternal aunt, age 60, alive and well.
- Maternal uncle, age 66, HTN.
- Paternal grandmother, age 87, HTN, cerebrovascular accident.
- Paternal grandfather, died of myocardial infarction at age 85.
- Paternal uncle, age 68, HTN.
- Paternal uncle, age 65, HTN.
- Denies family history of diabetes, kidney disease, allergies, asthma, drug or alcohol addiction, tuberculosis, bleeding disorders, or mental disorders.

Review of systems

General health status: No fever, chills, fatigue, depression, anxiety, or weight gain or loss this year. Says overall health is good. Weight has been stable for the last 5 years.

- **Integumentary:** No rashes, lesions, mole changes, or bruising.
- **HEENT:** No headaches, vision problems, hearing problems, sinus problems, frequent sore throats, or hoarseness.

Respiratory: No shortness of breath, wheezing, cough, productive cough, or history of tuberculosis.

Cardiovascular: No history of HTN, heart problems or murmurs, blood clots/phlebitis, chest pain, palpitations, edema, orthopnea, or claudication.

Gastrointestinal: No nausea/vomiting, abdominal pain, dysphagia, heartburn, jaundice, hemorrhoids, or blood in stool.

Genitourinary: No dysuria, frequency, urgency, penile discharge, or testicular masses; satisfied with sex life.

Musculoskeletal: No joint pains, swelling, or muscle weakness.

Neurological: No dizziness, vertigo, syncope, seizures, or numbness or tingling of extremities. History of a concussion in high school. Has never been treated for a mental disorder, depression, or anxiety.

Endocrine: No polyuria/polydipsia or heat or cold intolerance.

Lymphatic/hematological: No known exposure to hepatitis or other infectious disease; no cancer, bleeding, or anemia; has not had a blood transfusion.

Psychosocial profile

- **Self-care activities:** Does not seek routine health care screenings and has not had a physical examination in 2 years. Feels he is healthy and does not need to seek care unless he is sick or injured. Does not know his cholesterol level or usual BP. Does not know how to do TSE.

- **Typical day:** Arises at 4:30 a.m. Commutes to work and begins at 7:00 a.m. and works until 3:30 p.m. Drives home and relaxes, watches the news, and spends time with his family. He goes to bed by 10:00 p.m. each night.

- **Nutritional patterns:** Feels he eats a balanced diet, but evaluation reveals it is high in fats and cholesterol. Weight has been stable for last 5 years. 24 hour recall: Breakfast—8 oz. coffee with cream and 2 tsp sugar, 4 oz. orange juice, cream-filled donut. Lunch—Cheesesteak sandwich, French fries, and soda. Dinner—Fried chicken, mashed potatoes with butter, peas, salad with blue cheese dressing, 8 oz. glass of milk, and 8 oz. coffee with cream and 2 tsp of sugar, chocolate ice cream. Snack—Four chocolate chip cookies.

- **Activity/exercise patterns:** Work requires vigorous physical activity, including stair climbing, lifting, and repetitive motions. Sometimes plays basketball with friends on weekends.

- **Recreation/hobbies:** Enjoys watching sports on television and taking camping trips.

- **Sleep/rest patterns:** Sleeps well 7 to 8 hours a night and feels rested in the morning. Sometimes falls asleep watching television after dinner.

- **Personal habits:** Has six beers each weekend when watching sport programs. Has smoked five to eight cigarettes a day for the last 10 years. Denies recreational drug use.

- **Occupational health patterns:** States there are risks at work, but he takes full advantage of safety measures available.

- **Roles/relationships:** States he is in a good marriage that is supportive. States he is comfortable with his sexual relationship with his wife. Enjoys his children, especially his 5-year-old son.

- **Stress and coping:** Copes with problems by discussing them with wife. Often tries not to think about things that bother him.

- **Environmental health patterns:** Commute varies depending on location of current job, but is usually 30–50 miles/day. Usually wears seatbelt in car.

1. What would you include in Mr. Holsvick's physical assessment based on information provided in the health history?

2. What health education does the client need for his age, sex, and health risks?

_____

_____

Physical assessment findings

General appearance: A 32-year-old, well-developed, well-nourished, white man who appears stated age; no apparent distress at this time; moves all extremities well, gait normal. Dressed in work clothes and dusty.

- **Vital signs:** Temperature 97.9°F; pulse 68 beats/min; respirations 20/min; BP 138/86 mm Hg; height 5 feet, 9 inches; weight 170 lb.
- **Mental status:** Oriented to person, place, and time; appropriate affect; language well developed.
- **Integumentary:**
- Skin evenly colored, dry, without any worrisome lesions.
- Scar from work injury present on left lower leg.
- Hands dry with abrasions.
- Hair clean and thin.
- No clubbing present; positive capillary refill.
- **HEENT:**
- **Head/face:** Normocephalic; no lesions, tenderness, or masses; facial features symmetrical; no TMJ tenderness, locking, or clicking.
- **Eyes:**
- **Snellen:** R 20/25, L 20/20, both 20/20.
- Extraocular muscles intact, no nystagmus.
- Corneal light reflex symmetrical bilaterally.
- Visual fields normal by confrontation.
- Cornea and iris intact, anterior chamber clear.
- Sclera white, conjunctivae clear and glossy.
- PERRLA direct and consensual.
- Positive constriction and convergence.
- Red reflex present bilaterally, disks flat with sharp margins, vessels present without crossing defects, retina even color without hemorrhages or exudates, macula even-colored.
- **Ears:**
- External ear skin intact; no masses, lesions, or discharge.

- No tragus tenderness present.
- Webber test: No lateralization.
- Rhinne test: ac > bc.
- Whisper test normal.
- External ear canals clear without redness, swelling, lesions, or discharge.
- Tympanic membranes intact, pearly gray with light reflex and landmarks visible.
- **Nose:**
- Nares patent, no sinus tenderness present.
- Nasal mucosa pink.
- Septum intact, no deviation.
- **Mouth:**
- Lips, oral mucosa, and gingivae pink and moist without lesions.
- Teeth all present, clean, dental work present, no obvious caries.
- Pharynx pink, tonsils +1, palate intact.
- Tongue smooth, pink, symmetrical, no lesions.
- **Neck and axillae:**
- Thyroid not palpable.
- Carotid pulses +2 and equal. No bruits, no jugular venous distention.
- No lymphadenopathy of neck, axillae, or epitrochlear nodes.
- Trachea midline, no abnormal masses or pulsations.
- **Thorax:**
- S_1; S_2; no S_3, S_4, murmurs, gallops, or thrills present.
- PMI 1.5 cm at fifth ICS at midclavicular line.
- Anteroposterior less than transverse diameter, respiration unlabored.
- Chest expansion symmetrical; no tenderness, scars, masses, or lesions.
- Resonant percussion sound over lung fields.
- Lungs clear, no adventitious breath sounds heard.
- Breasts symmetrical; no masses, nipple discharge, or lymphadenopathy.

- Normal spinal curvatures with no tenderness.
- No costovertebral angle tenderness present.

Abdomen:

- Abdomen slightly rounded, positive respiratory movement, no masses or pulsations observed.
- Scar from previous surgery on right lower abdomen.
- Bowel sounds present, no vascular sounds heard.
- Tympany in all four quadrants.
- Abdomen soft, no hepatomegaly, liver 10 cm at the midclavicular line, no splenomegaly, no masses or tenderness
- No palpable lymph nodes in inguinal area.

Aorta 2 cm.

- No femoral bruits; pulses 2+ and equal.
- Musculoskeletal system and extremities:
- Joints and muscles symmetrical.
- Muscles well developed, +5 strength of upper and lower extremities.
- Full ROM of upper and lower extremities.
- Pulses 2+ bilaterally.
- DTRs 2+; positive plantar reflex.
- Skin warm, hair on both lower legs; no varicose veins; superficial and deep sensations intact.
- Gait normal, heel and toe walk and deep knee bend without difficulty, negative Romberg.

Genitalia:

- Circumcised male.

- External genitalia without discharge, lesions, or abnormalities.
- No scrotal swelling.
- Testes smooth without masses.
- No hernia present.

Rectum:

- Perianal area intact without hemorrhoids.
- Prostate smooth, firm, without masses +1.
- Rectal wall smooth without masses or tenderness.
- Stool brown and occult blood negative.

Significant findings that influence your plan of care:

- A 32-year-old white man who appears in no distress and in good health.
- Physical findings all normal.
- Smokes 5 to 8 cigarettes a day; drinks beer in moderation.
- Diet is high in fat and cholesterol.
- Father died of sudden cardiac death at age 69 and had HTN.
- Is unaware of his blood pressure or cholesterol level.
- Is exposed to environmental risks on the job, causing him to suffer three injuries in the last 5 years that needed treatment.
- Discusses problems with wife, but also states, "I try not to think about my problems."

3. List the positive and negative influences on Mr. Holsvick's health status at this time.

_____

_____

4. Cluster the supporting data for the following nursing diagnoses:
   a. Knowledge deficit related to health promotion activities.

_____

   b. Risk of injury related to high-risk work environment.

_____

5. Identify any additional nursing diagnoses for this client.

_____

_____

6. Name a collaborative nursing diagnosis for this client. Be specific about what the expected outcome of the diagnosis would include.

_____

_____

Chapter 21

Assessing the Mother-to-Be

Name: _____	**Date:** _____
Course: _____	**Instructor:** _____

1. Many changes occur during pregnancy as a result of hormone changes and fetal growth. Match the changes in the first column with the appropriate definition in the second column.

Changes	**Definition**
1. Chloasma	a. Increased salivation
2. Linea nigra	b. Nosebleeds
3. Striae gravidarum	c. Softening of cervix
4. Angioma	d. Craving unusual foods
5. Palmar erythema	e. Mask of pregnancy
6. Hirsutism	f. Heartburn
7. Epistaxis	g. Increased pigmentation of linea alba
8. Epulis	h. Increased hair growth
9. Ptyalism	i. Bluish discoloration of cervix
10. Pica	j. Separation of abdominal recti muscles
11. Pyrosis	k. Vascular spiders
12. Goodell's sign	l. Stretch marks
13. Chadwick's sign	m. Redness on palms of hands
14. Hegar's sign	n. Raised, red nodules on gums
15. Diastasis recti abdominis	o. Softening of uterus

2. Identify the following signs and symptoms as presumptive, probable, or positive of pregnancy.

   a. Fetal heart sounds _____

   b. Nausea _____

   c. Abdominal enlargement _____

   d. Breast tenderness _____

   e. Hegar's sign _____

   f. Chadwick's sign _____

   g. Skin changes _____

   h. Fatigue _____

   i. Positive pregnancy test _____

   j. Braxton-Hicks contractions _____

   k. Visualization of fetus by ultrasound _____

   l. Ballottement _____

   m. Frequent urination _____

   n. Quickening _____

   o. Amenorrhea _____

3. You are taking your client's health history. Name at least three diseases that are a cause for concern during pregnancy.

   _____

4. What additional assessments do you need to include in the prenatal assessment to monitor fetal development?

   _____

5. Your client's LMP was 10/1/02. Calculate the estimated date of confinement using Nägele's rule (LMP + 7 days − 3 months).

   _____

6. What should you include in the postpartum assessment?

   _____

   _____

7. When assessing a pregnant client, what changes or common findings might you see from head to toe?

   _____

   _____

8. Consider your own ethnic background. What, if any, cultural practices are associated with pregnancy and delivery?

   _____

   _____

Name: _____   Date: _____

Course: _____   Instructor: _____

Abnormal Case Study: Sara Silverstone

Sara Silverstone, age 28, is a married elementary school teacher, gravida 1, para 1. She delivered a 9-lb boy by cesarean section owing to failure to progress. Spinal duramorph anesthesia was administered. She is admitted to the maternity unit with an intravenous line of 5% dextrose in lactated Ringer's solution 125 mL/h infusing in her left hand. Because her condition is unstable, you perform a focused assessment.

Physical Assessment

- *General health status:* Temperature 99°F; awake, alert, oriented × 3; feels "wiped out" but happy.
- *Integumentary:* Skin color pale, nailbeds pale, capillary refill > 3 seconds, mucous membranes dry and pale, skin cool and clammy.
- *Respiratory:* Respirations 12/min and shallow.
- *Cardiovascular:* Tachycardia 118 beats/min and regular, BP 90/50 mm Hg, positive systolic murmur 2/6, + 2 pulses.

- *Breasts:* Firm, increased venous pattern, dark areolae, nipples everted, plans to breastfeed.
- *Abdomen:* Distended, dressings dry and intact, no bowel sounds, abdomen tender, uterus soft at umbilicus, bleeding heavy with clots.
- *Genitourinary:* Foley catheter draining clear yellow urine.
- *Musculoskeletal:* Upper extremities + 5/5 muscle strength, lower extremities weak and numb.
- *Neurological:* Lower extremities decreased sensation, "feel numb."

9. What assessment findings are cause for concern?

_____

10. What assessment findings may signal a hemorrhage?

_____

_____

11. What assessment data are related to anesthesia and should be closely monitored?

_____

12. What additional assessment data would be helpful in evaluating Mrs. Silverstone's fluid status?

_____

13. Considering that this client had a cesarean section, what additional system warrants close assessment?

_____

14. When Mrs. Silverstone's condition stabilizes, what additional assessment data will be needed to plan her care?

_____

_____

15. Cluster the supporting data for the following nursing diagnoses:

    a. Fluid volume deficit related to bleeding.

    _____

    _____

    b. Risk for impaired ventilation.

    _____

    c. Risk for infection.

    _____

    d. Risk for pain.

    _____

16. List any additional nursing diagnoses.

    _____

    _____

Chapter 22

Assessing the Newborn and Infant

| Name: _____ | Date: _____ |
| Course: _____ | Instructor: _____ |

1. The newborn has many findings that are apparent at birth but disappear shortly after birth or within the first year of life. Match the finding in the first column with the appropriate definition in the second column.

Findings	**Definition**
1. Acrocyanosis	a. Peeling of skin
2. Vernix caseosa	b. Small white, pearl-like epithelial cysts on palate
3. Desquamation	c. White cheesy substance on skin
4. Cutis marmorata	d. Dependent side of body red, nondependent side pale
5. Harlequin sign	e. Fine hair on face, back, and shoulders
6. Lanugo	f. Mottled skin
7. Milia	g. Hematoma between periosteum and skull
8. Epstein's pearls	h. Flat hemangioma at nape of neck
9. Craniosynostosis	i. Edema of soft scalp tissue from birth trauma
10. Stork bites	j. Premature closure of sutures
11. Caput succedaneum	k. Peripheral cyanosis
12. Cephalhematoma	l. White papules on face

2. What five areas are assessed with the Apgar score?

_____

3. What areas do you need to include in the newborn's health history?

   _____

4. What measurements should you include in your assessment of the newborn and infant?

   _____

5. Match the reflex in the first column to the proper technique in the second column.

Reflex	**Technique**
1. Moro	a. Tap gently on forehead
2. Startle	b. Place your finger in infant's palm
3. Tonic neck	c. Stroke side of face
4. Palmar	d. Suddenly jar crib or while holding infant in sitting position, let head drop back slightly
5. Plantar	e. Stroke lateral side of foot around to great toe
6. Babinski	f. Stroke lateral side of foot around to great toe
7. Stepping	g. Make a sudden loud noise
8. Crawling	h. With infant supine and leg extended, stimulate foot
9. Magnet	i. With infant prone, run fingers down sides of spine
10. Pull-to-sit	j. With leg flexed, apply pressure to sole of foot
11. Crossed extension	k. Place thumb against ball of foot
12. Trunk incurvation	l. With infant supine, turn head to one side
13. Rooting	m. Pull infant to sitting position
14. Sucking	n. Touch tip of infant's tongue
15. Extrusion	o. Touch infant's lip
16. Glabellar	p. Place infant on abdomen

6. When performing an assessment on a newborn or infant, what changes or common findings might you see from head to toe?

   _____

   _____

   _____

7. Consider your own ethnic background. What, if any, cultural practices are associated with care of the newborn?

   _____

   _____

Name: _____ Date: _____

Course: _____ Instructor: _____

Abnormal Case Study: Ryan Rogers

Martha Rogers, a 28-year-old, white, married woman, brings her 2-week-old son Ryan to the pediatrician's office. A full-term baby, Ryan had nursed well in the hospital, but now Mrs. Rogers is concerned. "Ryan's not keeping his feedings down," she states. "This is my first baby, and I'm afraid I must be doing something wrong." Ryan is lethargic and showing signs of dehydration. Considering the seriousness of his condition, you perform a focused assessment.

Health History

Chief complaint:

"Ryan's not keeping his feedings down."

Symptom analysis:

P—Vomits within an hour after feeding.
Q—"Vomits across the room." Vomit is stale milk.
R—After he vomits, he wants to nurse again as if he is hungry. He seems to be getting more lethargic.
S—At first, he vomited every now and then, but now he seems to vomit after every feeding.

T—Vomiting started when he was 1 week old.

Past health history:

- Pregnancy, labor, and delivery essentially uneventful.
- Apgar scores at birth 9/10, weight 8 lb.
- Began nursing right after delivery without problem.

Family history:

- Father had pyloric stenosis when he was 5 weeks old.

8. What factors in Ryan's history place him at risk for pyloric stenosis? Why?

_____

_____

_____

9. Because the risk for dehydration is a concern, what additional questions should you ask Mrs. Rogers that would give clues to Ryan's hydration status?

_____

_____

_____

Physical Assessment

- *General appearance:* Lethargic.
- *Vital signs:* Temperature 100°F, pulse 180 beats/min, respirations 45/min, weight 7 lb.
- *Integumentary:* Poor turgor, skin warm and dry.
- *HEENT:* Sunken fontanels, mucous membranes pink, but dry.
- *Respiratory:* Tachypnea, lungs clear.

- *Cardiovascular:* Tachycardia.
- *Abdomen:* Distended upper abdomen, visible reverse peristaltic waves in epigastric area, positive bowel sounds, palpable, olive-shaped mass in epigastric region.
- *Neurologicial/musculoskeletal:* Weak, responds to tactile stimuli, not very active.

10. Which assessment findings suggest pyloric stenosis?

_____

_____

11. Which assessment findings suggest dehydration?

_____

_____

12. Considering Ryan's age, what developmental tasks (Erikson) would be appropriate at this stage?

_____

13. Name one nursing intervention that would help Ryan maintain trust.

_____

14. Cluster the supporting data for the following nursing diagnoses:

    a. Fluid volume deficit related to vomiting.

    _____

    _____

    b. Altered nutrition less than body requirements related to inability to retain feedings.

    _____

15. The following diagnosis is potential or at risk for. State a possible reason for this diagnosis: risk for aspiration.

_____

16. Identify any additional nursing diagnoses for Ryan.

_____

_____

Chapter 23

Assessing the Toddler and Preschooler

Name: _____   Date: _____

Course: _____   Instructor: _____

1. The developmental task for the toddler is autonomy versus shame and doubt. What type of behaviors might you see if your client has been successful at this stage? What type of behaviors might you see if he or she has been unsuccessful at this stage?

_____

_____

_____

2. The developmental task for the preschooler is initiative versus guilt. What type of behaviors might you see if your client has been successful at this stage? What type of behaviors might you see if he or she has been unsuccessful at this stage?

_____

_____

3. What are the major health issues for the toddler and preschooler?

_____

4. Name six assessment findings that might lead you to suspect child abuse.

_____

_____

_____

5. What factors should you consider when performing a physical assessment on a toddler or preschooler?

_____

_____

6. How does the physical examination differ from an adult's examination?

_____

_____

7. When performing an assessment on a toddler or preschooler, what changes or common findings might you see from head to toe?

_____

_____

8. Consider your own ethnic background. What are your culture's expectations for children?

_____

Name: _____	Date: _____
Course: _____	Instructor: _____

Abnormal Case Study: Max Ingram

Max Ingram, age 15 months, is brought into the ED by his 17-year-old mother. She voices concern that he has a "high fever" and is chronically fussy and irritable. His admitting vital signs are as follows: temperature 101.2°F rectally, pulse 158 beats/min, respirations 32/min, and BP 112/74 mm Hg. Max weighs 20 lb and is 29.5 inches tall. He whines and clings to his mother throughout the history and physical examination, while she tries to get him to take a bottle of milk. You notice that besides his small size, his complexion is pale.

Health History

Biographical data:

- 15-month-old white boy with one younger sibling.
- Health insurance: medical card.
- Lives with single mother (17 years old, unemployed). Mother and children are living with a "good friend" at present until mother can find employment (friend's address provided and verified).

Current health status:

- Mother describes child's health as "okay" until past few months, when child developed increased fussiness, decreased activity tolerance, and trouble sleeping.
- Mother reports increased respiratory infections and claims child "feels feverish a lot." Is unable to be specific regarding circumstances (does not have thermometer).

Past health history:

- No prenatal care until third trimester; forceps delivery with epidural after 18-hour labor.
- Infant born "a few weeks early" but went home with mother at discharge; unsure of Apgar score; reports infant cried at birth and fed without difficulty.

- Hospitalized for respiratory syncytial virus at 6 months; treated for three episodes of otitis media in first year (unsure of dates/age of infant at time). Claims he has "lots of colds."
- Has not had immunizations beyond his "second set after he was born."
- No medications other than antibiotics; gives Tylenol if "feverish" or fussy; has given "purple" OTC cold medication (unsure of name).
- Denies known allergies to medications, but thinks child has allergies or asthma.

Family history:

- Mother describes her health as "good." Says she "gets colds once or twice a year."
- Maternal grandfather left family when mother was 8 years old; health unknown.
- Maternal grandmother's health "poor" secondary to arthritis and "mental problems."
- Mother reports her three older siblings are in "good" health.
- Child's father's health "good" as far as is known. Mother does not maintain contact with him (same father for both children).
- Paternal grandfather died in auto accident in his 30s—no known health problems.
- Paternal grandmother is in her 60s and has diabetes mellitus.
- Multiple paternal siblings—health unknown.

Review of systems:

- *General health status:* More fussy and irritable than usual, more colds than usual, sleeping poorly.

- *Integumentary:* Denies changes in skin, hair, or nails.

- *HEENT:* Tugs at ears; denies hoarseness, rubbing eyes, or excessive tearing/redness.

- *Respiratory:* More frequent colds.

- *Cardiovascular:* Can feel "heart racing and pounding in his chest," especially with crying/exertion.

- *Gastrointestinal:* Occasional diarrhea/vomiting that never lasts beyond 1 day.

- *Genitourinary:* Circumcised, urinates without difficulty.

- *Musculoskeletal:* Denies difficulties/concerns.

- *Neurological:* Denies seizure-like activity, feels child hears and sees okay.

- *Lymphatic:* More frequent episodes of colds; worries it's because he's behind on shots.

Psychosocial profile:

- *Self-care activities:* Holds own bottle, feeds self, indicates wants by pointing/fussing.

- *Nutritional patterns:* Switched to "regular milk" (unsure if whole) at about 10–11 months for convenience and because less expense. Child still drinks from bottle—about eight 8-oz. bottles per day. "Picky eater but loves milk." Occasionally eats toast, applesauce, cereal. Seldom offers water because child usually refuses. Mother not concerned about weight because she was "tiny" as a child. *24-Hour dietary recall:* Breakfast—8 oz. milk, $\frac{1}{4}$ cup applesauce. Midmorning—>8 oz. milk. Lunch—$\frac{1}{4}$ cup Ramen noodles without broth, >8 oz. milk. Afternoon—8-oz. milk bottle for nap, 8 oz. Pepsi on awakening. Supper— Refused pizza, >8 oz. milk, cookie. Bedtime—8 oz. milk for bedtime. Mother claims this is fairly typical, usually eats a little more but appetite has diminished. Occasionally wants bottle if awakens at night.

- *Activity/exercise patterns:* Says he is not an active child. Prefers to play quietly and spends most time indoors watching TV. Describes him as quiet and slow to warm up to people but generally a "good baby."

- *Elimination:* Still in diapers, has semisolid light brown bowel movement daily or less, denies constipation, has occasional diarrhea/vomiting.

- *Sleep/rest patterns:* Sleeps about 8–10 hours per night with two or three daytime naps lasting 1–3 hours. Gives bottle to help sleep; puts child to bed abut 9 p.m. (denies routine), and child spontaneously awakens about 7 or 8 a.m. and plays quietly until mother gets him up around 9 a.m. Usually sleeps "okay" with occasional awakening but self-soothes back to sleep; more fussy past few months when awakening at night.

- *Personal habits:* Starting to put things in mouth, including dirt and small debris he finds on floor. Mother smokes about 10–20 cigarettes a day. Child permitted to have soft drinks—limits to one bottle of soda per day because she feels more would not be good for him.

- *Occupational health patterns:* Child is dependent on mother for needs. Mother applied for assistance about 3 months ago but has not followed up. Mother did not finish high school; claims she wants to find a job, but unless she can find affordable and accessible child care, she is limited in what she does and where she works.

- *Environmental health patterns:* Family lives in "very old house" with peeling paint and loose plaster, but mother denies noticing if child ingests any. Has tried to ensure that cleaning supplies and medications are kept out of child's reach. Stairways are open, but child "ignores them" or stays away if she yells at him. Lives on busy street, so child usually is kept inside, although there is a small, fenced backyard where child occasionally plays. Friend's car is equipped with seatbelts, which they don't use, and children do not have car safety seats.

- *Roles/relationships:* Mother claims to have loving relationship with child. Child described as a "good baby" who does not give her "much grief." Child's father never lived with family and has no contact. Family currently lives with male friend of mother's. Mother claims he gets along with her children "okay" and denies abuse/violence. No contact with maternal relatives except child's aunt (mother's older sister), who sometimes helps them with money and clothes.

- *Stress and coping:* Child cries/fusses when uncomfortable or upset. Mother soothes him with a bottle or will give Tylenol (assumes he feels bad); disciplines by smacking hands or telling "no." Child is usually compliant and seldom has to be spanked/scolded.

9. What information from the health history indicates that Max is at risk for a nutritional deficiency?

   _____

10. What information from the 24-hour dietary recall indicates a nutritional deficiency?

   _____

11. What factors from Max's history increase his risk for an ear infection?

   _____

   _____

12. Aside from the nutritional deficit, what other health problems is Max at risk for?

   _____

Physical Assessment

- *General appearance:* Generally passive/withdrawn; whimpers and clings to mother with no vigorous objection to health care providers; pale, sits limply in mother's lap; appears small for age.
- *Vital signs:* Temperature 101.2°F (rectal); pulse 158 beats/min; respirations 32/min; full/deep; BP 112/74 mm Hg; weight 20 lb, height 29.5 inches.
- *Integumentary:* Skin warm and moist; nails spoon-shaped, brittle.
- *HEENT:*
- Normocephalic with fine, evenly distributed hair; scalp dry/flaky.
- Pupils equal, responsive to light; light reflexes equal; follows object through all fields; sclerae white, conjunctivae pale.
- Dirty behind ears; scant light brown cerumen bilaterally; tympanic membranes bulging and red with little mobility.
- Nose aligned midline, no septal deviation, membranes pale/moist.
- Dentition present and showing signs of decay consistent with prolonged bottle feeding; tongue midline, gag intact; throat pink, without exudate/erythema.
- Mild lymphadenopathy.
- *Respiratory:* Rate 32/min and labored, breath sounds equal bilaterally, clear to auscultation; mild grunting.
- *Cardiovascular:* Marked precordial pulsation; point of maximal impulse readily visible and palpable lateral to midclavicular line in sixth ICS; rate 158 beats/min, regular
- *Gastrointestinal:* Bowel sounds present, regular, although slightly diminished; no signs of distress with palpation; no palpable masses.
- *Genitourinary:* Normal male genitalia; meatus midline and nonerythematous, testes descended bilaterally; anus normal.
- *Musculoskeletal:* Minimal muscle resistance; full passive ROM; extremities symmetrical, no joint swelling/inflammation; stands and walks to return to mother; gait normal for age.
- *Neurological:* Cranial nerves intact; DTRs equal/diminished; developmentally delayed.

13. What assessment findings suggest that Max may have another ear infection?

_____

14. What assessment findings suggest that Max may have anemia?

_____

15. Max's mother says she can feel his heart racing and pounding in his chest. What might account for the marked precordial pulsation and rapid heart rate?

_____

16. Identify teaching needs for Max's mother.

_____

17. Considering Max's age, what developmental tasks (Erikson) would be appropriate at this stage?

_____

18. Name one developmental task for this developmental stage.

_____

19. Cluster the supporting data for the following nursing diagnosis:

    a. Altered nutrition less than body requirements related to poor dietary intake.

    _____

20. The following diagnoses are potential or at risk for. State a possible reason for each diagnosis:

    a. Potential complication: hyperthermia related to infection.

    _____

    b. Risk for infection related to increased susceptibility.

    _____

    c. Risk for injury.

    _____

21. Identify any additional nursing diagnoses for Max.

    _____

    _____

Chapter 24

Assessing the School-Age Child and Adolescent

Name: _____	**Date:** _____
Course: _____	**Instructor:** _____

1. The developmental task for the school-age child is industry versus inferiority. What type of behavior might you see if your client has been successful at this stage? What type of behavior might you see if he or she has been unsuccessful at this stage?

   _____

   _____

2. The developmental task for the adolescent is identity versus role diffusion. What type of behavior might you see if your client has been successful at this stage? What type of behavior might you see if he has been unsuccessful at this stage?

   _____

   _____

3. What health concerns should you screen for during your assessment?

   _____

4. Identify areas of health teaching for school-age and adolescent clients.

   _____

5. How does the physical examination differ from an adult's?

   _____

   _____

6. When assessing a school-age child or adolescent, what changes or common findings might you see from head to toe?

_____

_____

7. Consider your ethnic background. What is your culture's expectation for adolescents?

_____

Name: _____	*Date:* _____
Course: _____	*Instructor:* _____

Abnormal Case Study: Nathan Lyons

Nathan Lyons, age 10, is admitted to the hospital with acute lymphocytic leukemia. His mother states that he was fine until a few weeks ago, when he began complaining that he was tired all the time. He also noticed that his gums bled when he brushed his teeth and that he had bruises on his arms but couldn't remember hurting them.

Health History

Chief complaint:

"I'm tired all the time."

Symptom analysis:

P—No precipitating event, some relief with rest.
Q—"Just tired, no energy."
R—Related signs/symptoms include bleeding gums and bruising.
S—Seems to be getting worse.
T—Started a few weeks ago.

Past health history:

- Frequent ear infections until age 6.
- No surgeries, hospitalizations, or trauma.
- Immunizations up-to-date.
- Allergies: no known drug allergies; has had penicillin without reaction, no food or environmental allergies.
- No medications.

Family history:

- Family history of leukemia.

Review of systems:

- *General health status:* Fatigue, loss of appetite, weight loss of a couple of pounds in the past month.
- *Integumentary:* Unexplained bruising.
- *HEENT:* Bleeding gums, "lumps" in neck.
- *Respiratory:* Shortness of breath with activity.
- *Cardiovascular:* No complaints.
- *Musculoskeletal:* Weakness.
- *Neurological:* No complaints.

Psychosocial profile:

- *Health patterns/beliefs:* Always has annual checkup. Mother says, "I always try to be proactive."
- *Typical day:* Awakens at 7 a.m., has breakfast, leaves for school by 8 a.m. Has classes until 3 p.m.; participates in after-school sports until 5 p.m. Dinner at 6 p.m., homework 7 to 9 p.m.; then takes shower and goes to bed by 10 p.m. Does well in school.
- *Nutritional patterns: 24-hour recall:* Breakfast—4 oz. orange juice, cereal with milk. Lunch—Peanut butter and jelly sandwich, cookies, milk. Snack—Fruit snack and milk. Dinner—Hamburger, French fries, chocolate cake.
- *Sleep/rest patterns:* Sleeps 9 hours uninterrupted.
- *Activity/exercise patterns:* Loves sports, uses protective equipment.
- *Environmental health patterns:* Home environment has safety alarms and smoke detectors; lives in suburbs.
- *Religious/cultural influences:* Protestant; English heritage, no cultural influence on health.
- *Social supports:* Family, school friends.

Physical Assessment

- *General appearance:* Awake, alert, oriented × 3, color pale, looks tired.
- *Vital signs:* Temperature 99°F, pulse 104 beats/min, respirations 22/min, BP 100/60 mm Hg.
- *Integumentary:* Skin color pale, mucous membranes and conjunctiva pale, several bruises (3 cm) noted on arms bilaterally, no other lesions.

- *HEENT:* Gums bleeding, positive cervical lymphadenopathy.
- *Respiratory:* Lungs clear.
- *Cardiovascular:* heart regular rate and rythm, tachycardia, systolic murmur II/VI.
- *Abdomen*: Positive splenomegaly and hepatomegaly.
- *Musculoskeletal/neurological:* Able to move all extremities, but generalized weakness.

8. Identify the assessment data that may indicate anemia or bleeding.

_____

_____

9. Identify the assessment data that may indicate infection.

_____

10. Considering anemia, bleeding, and infection are common complications of acute lymphocytic leukemia, identify pertinent nursing diagnoses.

_____

_____

_____

11. Cluster the supporting data for the following nursing diagnoses:

   a. Altered nutrition less than body requirements.

   _____

   b. Fatigue related to inadequate tissue perfusion secondary to anemia.

   _____

12. Identify any additional nursing diagnoses for Nathan.

_____

13. Considering Nathan's age, what developmental tasks (Erikson) would be appropriate at this stage?

_____

14. Identify a developmental task for this stage of development.

_____

Name: _____	Date: _____
Course: _____	Instructor: _____

Abnormal Case Study: Sally Randolph

Sally Randolph, age 18, presents to your clinic complaining of amenorrhea for 7 months. Sally is a college freshman on a track athletic scholarship. She says she is usually healthy, has no other symptoms, and has not lost weight. She exercises daily by running 12 miles in the morning at 6:00 a.m. and 12 miles in the evening at 6:00 p.m., and she eats three meals a day. She comes from a large farm family, is the oldest of 5 children, and is the first in her family to go to college. She has been a track athlete for 2 years.

Health History

Chief complaint:

"I'm worried because I haven't had my period in 7 months, and I want to find out if something is wrong."

Current health status

- No recent weight loss.
- Denies problems with appetite, has a healthy diet, denies anorexia or bulimia symptoms.
- Denies being sexually active.
- Before amenorrhea, her periods were light and lasted for about 5 days.

15. Considering Sally's history, what first comes to mind as a contributing factor to her amenorrhea?

Past health history:

- Menarche age 16.
- Has never been sexually active and has never used oral contraceptives.
- Has never sustained any physical trauma.
- Has never had surgery.
- Was anemic, but it was 1 year ago.
- Only medication she takes is a multivitamin.
- Has never had a gynecological examination.
- No history of vaginal or reproductive organ infections.

Family history:

- Both parents alive and well.
- Three younger brothers and one younger sister, all healthy.

Psychosocial profile:

- *Nutritional/weight patterns:* Good appetite, eats at least three meals a day, no recent weight gain or loss, fluid intake exceeds 2 L/day.
- *Activity/exercise patterns:* Runs 12 miles every morning and evening year round. Rarely does any other form of exercise.
- *Sleep/rest patterns:* Sleeps about 7 hours each night.
- *Personal habits:* Does not drink alcohol or use tobacco products.
- *Environmental health patterns:* Lives in college residence hall with one roommate; first time away from home for more than 1 week; comes from small farming community.

16. Considering the age of menarche for Sally, how else might you explain her amenorrhea?

_____

_____

17. Would this amenorrhea be considered primary or secondary?

_____

_____

Physical Assessment

- *General appearance:* Appears younger than 18 years; affect is appropriate; she is communicative and willing to undergo examination.
- *Height:* 5 feet, 1 inch.
- *Weight:* 100 lb.

Inspection:

- *Integumentary:* Hair distribution appropriate for maturational level.
- *Genitalia:* No lesions, other signs of infection, or obvious congenital abnormalities.
- Cervix is midline, clear, and pink and without lesions; os is patent.

Palpation:

- *Genitalia:* No swelling or induration of labia, urethral meatus, Skene's glands, or Bartholin's gland. Vaginal muscle tone strong.
- *Bimanual:* Cervix mobile, nontender; uterus small, pear-shaped, firm, mobile, nontender, anteverted.
- *Adnexa:* Ovaries firm bilaterally, mobile, and nontender.

18. Aside from amenorrhea, are there any other findings that warrant further investigation?

_____

_____

19. Considering Sally's age, what developmental tasks (Erikson) would be appropriate at this stage?

_____

_____

20. Identify a developmental task for this stage of development.

_____

_____

21. The following diagnoses are potential or at risk for. State the reasoning for each possible diagnosis:

   a. Risk for altered nutritional pattern less than bodily requirements.

   _____

   _____

   b. Risk for altered health maintenance related to inadequate understanding of exercise and menstrual cycle.

   _____

   _____

22. Identify any additional nursing diagnoses.

_____

_____

_____

Chapter 25

Assessing the Older Adult

Name: _____	**Date:** _____
Course: _____	**Instructor:** _____

1. Identify three factors that may confuse symptoms reported by older adults.

   _____

   _____

2. What might you do differently when obtaining a history from an older client?

   _____

   _____

3. The developmental task for the older client is integrity versus despair. What type of behavior might you see if your client has been successful at this stage? What type of behavior might you see if he or she has been unsuccessful at this stage?

   _____

   _____

4. List five factors that you should consider when performing a physical assessment on an older client.

   _____

   _____

5. When performing an assessment on an older client, what changes might you see from head to toe?

   _____

   _____

6. Match the types of incontinence in the first column with the definitions in the second column.

Types of Incontinence	Definitions
1. Stress	a. Urine leakage resulting from inability to get to bathroom because of cognitive or physical impairment
2. Urge	b. Involuntary loss of urine with increased intra-abdominal pressure
3. Overflow	c. Leakage of urine resulting from inability to delay voiding
4. Functional	d. Leakage of urine from an overdistended bladder

7. Consider your ethnic background. What is your culture's view of the role of the older adult in the family and in society? How is the older adult cared for?

Name: _____	*Date:* _____
Course: _____	*Instructor:* _____

Abnormal Case Study: Arthur O'Reilly

Arthur O'Reilly, age 65, has DJD and is being admitted to the orthopedic unit for total knee replacement. A retired floor installer and refinisher, the client lives with wife and has a 30-year-old son who lives nearby.

Health History

Chief complaint:

"The pain in my knee is getting worse, and I can hardly get around."

Symptom analysis:

P—Pain with activity, pain is worse when the weather is bad, some relief with rest and medication.
Q—Dull, aching persistent pain.
R—Knees.
S—8/10, unrelenting.
T—started 5 years ago.

Past health history:

- Had measles, mumps, chickenpox, and rubella but unable to remember specifics.
- Inguinal hernia repair at age 45, torn medial collateral ligaments at age 50, no hospitalizations.
- History of HTN.
- No known drug allergies; has had penicillin without reaction; no food or environmental allergies.
- Nonsteroidal anti-inflammatory drugs (celecoxib [Celebrex]) for arthritis; furosemide (Lasix), 20 mg once daily, for HTN.

Family history:

Family history of HTN, cardiovascular disease, and DJD.

Review of systems:

- *General health status:* Usually feels okay except when knee is hurting.
- *Integumentary:* No reported problems.
- *HEENT:* No reported problems.
- *Respiratory:* No reported problems.
- *Cardiovascular:* No chest pain or palpitations; last ECG 1 year ago and normal.
- *Genitourinary:* No reported problems.
- *Musculoskeletal:* Weakness in lower extremities, difficulty walking.
- *Neurological:* No reported problems.

Psychosocial profile:

- *Health patterns and beliefs/self-care activities:* Usually sees physician only when sick, but is seen every few months for HTN.
- *Typical day:* Awakens at 7 a.m., eats breakfast with wife, reads paper, works in garden until lunch, takes nap in afternoon, has dinner, watches TV until 11 p.m., and goes to bed.
- *Activity/exercise patterns:* Not as active as usual because of knee pain; has to use a cane.
- *Sleep/rest patterns:* Usually gets 7–8 hours of sleep a night, but awakens at times with knee pain.
- *Occupational health patterns:* Retired.
- *Roles, relationships, self-concept:* Married 32 years; says he feels like a "cripple."
- *Cultural/religious influences:* Irish Catholic; goes to church several times a week.

- *Sexuality patterns:* Knee pain sometimes affects sexual activity.
- *Social supports:* Wife and son are major sources of support. Has been married for 32 years.

Physical Assessment
- *General appearance:* Well-developed, obese man; appears stated age. Responds appropriately, affect pleasant. Ambulates with cane.
- *Vital signs:* Temperature 98.6°F, pulse 80 beats/min, respirations 18/min, BP 150/90 mm Hg, height 6 feet, weight 250 lb.
- *Integumentary:* Skin intact, warm, dry, and pink; several seborrhea keratosis lesions on upper torso.
- *HEENT:*
- Head: Symmetrical midline.
- Eyes: Vision 20/20 with corrective lenses, extraocular muscles intact, peripheral vision intact, funduscopic examination within normal limits.
- Ears: Hearing intact, tympanic membrane intact and pearly gray, no drainage.
- Nose: Patent, no drainage.
- Mouth and throat: Mucous membranes pink, moist, and intact, no lesions; has upper partial bridge.
- *Respiratory:* Lungs clear.
- *Cardiovascular:* Regular rate and rhythm (heart regular rate and rhythm) +S_4, +2 pulses.
- *Abdomen:* Large and round, soft, nontender, positive bowel sounds, no organomegaly.
- *Musculoskeletal:* Full ROM of upper extremities, decreased ROM of knees, positive crepitus and swelling, +4/5 muscle strength lower extremities, +5/5 upper extremities.
- *Neurological:* Awake, alert, oriented × 3, gait unsteady related to DJD, CN I–XII intact, sensory intact, +2 DTRs.

8. Considering Mr. O'Reilly's age, what developmental tasks (Erikson) would be appropriate at this stage?

_____

9. How might Mr. O'Reilly's illness affect his ability to be successful at this stage of development?

_____

10. Mr. O'Reilly has DJD. How does this differ from rheumatoid arthritis?

_____

11. From Mr. O'Reilly's history, identify risk factors for DJD.

_____

12. From Mr. O'Reilly's physical assessment findings, identify signs of DJD.

_____

_____

13. Cluster the supporting data for the following nursing diagnoses.

    a. Pain related to physical activity.

    _____

    b. Impaired physical mobility related to pain and weakness.

    _____

    c. Sleep pattern disturbance related to pain.

    _____

14. Identify any additional nursing diagnoses for Mr. O'Reilly.

    _____

    _____

Answers

Some questions may have additional answers. Check the appropriate chapter in the text.

Chapter 1: Health Assessment and the Nurse

1.

Nausea: Subjective

Cyanosis: Objective

Jaundice: Objective

Edema: Objective

Numbness: Subjective

Diaphoresis: Objective

Pallor: Objective

Ptosis: Objective

Dizziness: Subjective

Stridor: Objective

Palpitations: Subjective

Irregular pulse: Objective

Shortness of breath: Subjective

Chest pain: Subjective

2.

a. Lauren

b. Mother, old records

c. "My ear hurts" and irritable

d. 2-year-old girl with 103°F temperature, cough, runny nose, decreased sleep and oral intake, tugging at ear, history of otitis media × 3

3.

1. c

2. f

3. g

4. h

5. b

6. d

7. a

8. e

4.

   a. "What does it feel like, and when did it start? Point to where it hurts."

   b. "Would you like to talk about this?"

   c. "What makes you feel this way? Would you like to talk about it?"

   d. "What has your doctor said?"

   e. "I'm here now. How can I help you?"

5.

Communication Problem	Correct Question/Statement
a. Leading client	"Can you point to where it hurts?"
b. Giving advice	"What do you feel is best?"
c. Offering false reassurance	"You seem concerned, would you like to talk about it?"
d. Using medical jargon	"You're going to have your ovaries removed through a laparoscope. The doctor will make a couple of small incisions…"
e. Using clichés	"Would you like to talk about this?"
f. Asking more than one question at a time	"What seems to be the problem?"
g. Taking responses personally	"I can see that you're upset. How can I help you?"
h. Changing the subject	"Would you like to talk about this?"
i. Assuming	Review the entire preoperative phase with your client regardless of his or her educational level.
j. Feeling uncomfortable with subject	"Would you like to talk about this?"
k. Assuming rather than clarifying	"Was there a problem with taking your medications?"

6.

   a. Rose Montefalco

   b. Old records

   c. "My chest is killing me; it feels like I'm in a vice." Pain severity 10/10, down to 8/10 after nitroglycerin administration; difficulty breathing.

   d. BP 170/110 mm Hg; pulse 118 beats/min, regular; respirations 32/min; temperature 99.8°F; pulse oximetry 90% on room air; cardiac monitor shows sinus tachycardia with occasional premature ventricular contractions. BP 160/100 mm Hg; pulse 110 beats/min; respirations 28/min; pulse oximetry 93% on 3 L of oxygen after nitroglycerin.

7.

S—"My chest is killing me; it feels like I'm in a vice."

O—78-year-old woman; BP 170/110 mm Hg; pulse 118 beats/min, regular; respirations 32/min; temperature 99.8°F; pulse oximetry 90% on room air. Monitor shows sinus tachycardia with occasional premature ventricular contractions. Diaphoretic, pale, and clammy.

A—Chest pain, altered cardiovascular status, and ineffective breathing.

P—Relieve pain, establish effective breathing, and stabilize cardiovascular status.

I—Continue to monitor, obtain diagnostic test results, titrate nitroglycerin, continue oxygen.

E—Vital signs more stable, pulse oximetry 93% on 3 L of oxygen, chest pain 8/10.

8.

D—"My chest is killing me…"; 78-year-old woman; BP 170/110 mm Hg; pulse 118 beats/min, regular; respirations 32/min; temperature 99.8°F; pulse oximetry 90% on room air. Monitor shows sinus tachycardia with occasional premature ventricular contractions. Diaphoretic, pale, and clammy.

A—Oxygen at 3 L, cardiac monitor, intravenous nitroglycerin, obtain diagnostic tests.

R—Chest pain 8/10 after start of nitroglycerin; BP 160/100 mm Hg; pulse 110 beats/min; respirations 28/min; pulse oximetry 93% on 3 L of oxygen.

9.

P—Chest pain, ineffective breathing, altered cardiovascular status.

I—Oxygen at 3 L; intravenous nitroglycerin; continue cardiac monitoring; obtain diagnostic tests.

E—Chest pain 8/10 after intravenous nitroglycerin; BP 160/100 mm Hg; pulse 110 beats/min; respirations 28/min; pulse oximetry 93% on 3 L of oxygen.

10.

Not specific

11.

1
1
3
3
2

Chapter 2: The Health History

1.

a. Biographical data
b. Biographical data
c. Family history
d. Current health status
e. Biographical data
f. Psychosocial profile
g. Past health history
h. Psychosocial profile
i. Review of systems
j. Past health history
k. Review of systems
l. Past health history

    m. Current health status

    n. Psychosocial profile

    o. Review of systems

    p. Biographical data

    q. Review of systems

    r. Biographical data

    s. Psychosocial profile

    t. Review of systems

    u. Psychosocial profile

    v. Review of systems

    w. Biographical data

    x. Psychosocial profile

    y. Review of systems

2.

1. e
2. a
3. b
4. c
5. g
6. h
7. f
8. d

Chapter 3: Approach to the Physical Assessment

1.

1. d
2. e
3. a
4. b
5. c
6. k
7. j
8. l
9. f
10. h
11. i
12. g

2.

    a. Bimanual palpation

    b. Palpation

    c. Percussion

    d. Inspection

    e. Auscultation

    f. Palpation

    g. Ballottement

    h. Ballottement

    i. Fist percussion

    j. Percussion

    k. Auscultation

    l. Palpation

3.

    a. Balls or ulnar surface

    b. Dorsal part

    c. Finger pads/tips

4.

The difference in weight and subsequent thickness of the chest wall may account for the difference in breath sounds, although both are normal. When assessing for abnormalities, use the client as his or her own comparative.

5.

Infants: Have parent hold infant; do otoscopic and funduscopic examinations last.

Preschoolers: Have parent present; use toys, games, or demonstrate on dolls.

Adolescents: Ask if they want parent present (may be modest and say no).

Pregnant clients: Assess mother and fetus; include fundal height and fetal heart tone.

Older adults: Avoid certain examination positions if client has trouble assuming them; allow for vision and hearing deficits.

6.

    a. Lithotomy or dorsal recumbent

    b. Flexed at hips leaning over table

    c. Supine

    d. Standing

    e. Sitting

    f. Supine or sitting

    g. Sims's or flexed at hips leaning over

7.

    a. High

    b. High

    c. Low

    d. Low

    e. High

8.

Cast or injury to arm, intravenous access, side of mastectomy, vascular access

9.

All systems are related, so they can affect or be affected by every system. If a problem occurs in one system, you may see changes in other systems, or vice versa.

Chapter 4: Teaching the Client

1.

Educational level, financial resources, and current health status (e.g., pain, age, stress, and available supports)

2.

Vision, hearing, cognitive ability, motor skills, breathing problems, and muscle strength

3.

Obesity, HTN, NIDDM, diet, noncompliance with taking prescribed medications

4.

Independent, has full-time job with medical insurance coverage, has supportive family

5.

    a. BP 180/100 mm Hg; glucose 160 mg/dL; overweight with poor diet; urinary signs and symptoms; missed medications; inconsistent glucose monitoring; jokes during examination; thinks she has a urinary tract infection and needs antibiotic so she can get back to work.

    b. Missed medications; inconsistent glucose monitoring; overweight with poor diet; jokes during examination; thinks she has a urinary tract infection and needs antibiotic so she can get back to work.

6.

The plan has to fit in with her work schedule.

Chapter 5: Assessing Wellness

1.

Supports: Family, friends, organized groups.

Psychological state: Client not only needs the information, but also needs to believe that it is important. Depression, anxiety, or stress may also affect health behaviors.

2.

Barriers to health care: Lack of money; lack of transportation; distant location of health care; and ethnic, gender, or age discrimination.

3.

Exercising right before bedtime may make it difficult to fall asleep.

Nicotine increases the time needed to fall asleep and causes lighter sleep.

Caffeine increases sleep latency and decreases total sleep time.

Alcohol affects the rapid-eye-movement sleep cycle and fragments sleep.

Obesity increases the risk for sleep apnea. Gaining weight increases sleep, and losing weight decreases sleep.

High-protein foods increase alertness; high-carbohydrate foods increase relaxation.

Stress decreases the ability to sleep.

Congestive heart failure can cause nocturnal dyspnea; pain associated with surgery can interrupt sleep.

4.

1. c
2. a
3. e
4. f
5. b
6. d

5.

Maximum = 145, Minimum = 87, Ideal = 116

6.

Infant: Unmet basic needs

Toddler: Separation from parents (e.g., owing to hospitalization)

School-age child: School

Adolescent: Physical changes of puberty; sexuality

Young adult: Relationships and work

Middle-aged adult: Family and finances

Older adult: Retirement, illness, and finances

7.

Infant: Choking, accidental poisoning

Preschool/school-age child: Accidents related to bikes, sports

Adolescent: Accidents related to driving; health problems related to drugs or sex

Young adult/middle-aged adult: Work-related injuries

Older adult: Falls

Chapter 6: Assessing Nutrition

1.

1. c
2. a
3. e
4. b
5. d
6. g
7. f

2.

Excess water-soluble vitamins are excreted from the body. Fat-soluble vitamins are not excreted, so they can build up to toxic levels.

3.

- Vitamin A: Fat-soluble
- Vitamin B: Water-soluble
- Vitamin C: Water-soluble
- Vitamin D: Fat-soluble
- Vitamin E: Fat-soluble
- Vitamin K: Fat-soluble

4.

Infant/toddler: Fats for nervous system development

Preschool: Iron to prevent iron-deficiency anemia (common in this age group)

School-age child: Calcium for prepubertal bone development

Adolescent: Iron for girls to prevent anemia resulting from menstruation; calcium for bone development

Pregnant woman: Increased calories, milk, fluids, and vitamins (especially iron and folic acid) for fetal development

Older adult: Calcium to decrease risk for osteoporosis, especially in postmenopausal women; decreased calories to prevent obesity, an increased risk in this age group

8.

Cancer is always a possibility when an older client presents with unexplained weight loss. Because weight loss is a symptom of prostate cancer, rule this out first. Mr. Liang does not describe symptoms consistent with prostate concerns of any type, however. He himself has provided an important perspective on his weight loss—he says he doesn't like American food.

9.

Diet lacking in dairy and in all other food groups; deficit in fluid intake

10.

Inadequate diet and dehydration

11.

Digital rectal examination of the prostate and prostate-specific antigen test.

12.

Urinary complaints; enlarged, irregular, hard prostate; possible changes in bowel habits; possible back pain; and positive inguinal nodes if metastatic

13.

Fatigue, diet and loss of appetite, low BP, increased pulse and respirations, pale conjunctiva, positive systolic murmur 2/6, and low hematocrit and hemoglobin

14.

Approximate percent weight loss is 17%; approximate BMI is 16.2 (underweight).

15.

   a. Weight loss of 30 lb over 4–5 months, change in diet, and decreased appetite
   b. 24 oz. of fluid/day; skin dry and flaky; fatigue; low BP; increased pulse and respirations; and voids four times a day, concentrated yellow urine
   c. Complaints of increasing fatigue

Chapter 7: Spirituality Assessment

1.

Behavior: Praying
Communication: Talking about God
Relationships: Visits by clergy
Environment: Religious objects such as a rosary, Bible, or Koran

2.

Treatment, organ donation, abortion, dietary restrictions, gender of practitioner, and healing practices or rituals

3.

Dietary constraints (e.g., Kosher diet)

4.

Pro-life (antiabortion) viewpoint

5.

May want same-sex practitioner; women may want to keep head covered; may refuse treatment because of fatalistic view

6.

May wish to set up a small shrine in hospital room

7.

May wish to use a crystal for healing potential

8.

Mexican health practices encourage the use of a healer known as a curandero. Be aware of treatments prescribed by the healer, and evaluate them for any interactions with the client's medical regimen.

9.

People of Mexican heritage (usually Roman Catholic) often accept illness as a punishment from God for past sins. This belief may interfere with their seeking medical help or following a medical regimen. The client's priest may help facilitate compliance with medical treatments.

10.

She appears anxious and withdrawn, but when she speaks she says that her illness is a punishment. The religious symbols in her home and her use of rosary beads show that her spiritual life is important to her; however, she is in spiritual distress at present. You may need to assess further and intervene to help Mrs. Ramirez feel less anxious and more accepting of her illness and its treatment. Be sure to include the parish priest and her husband in your plan.

Chapter 8: Assessing the Integumentary System

1.

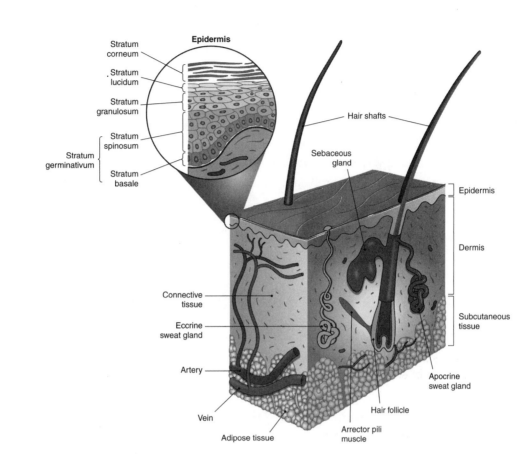

2.

1. c
2. n
3. f
4. o
5. g
6. j
7. h
8. l
9. k
10. m
11. a
12. i
13. b
14. e
15. d

3.

Central cyanosis: Inspect oral mucosa or conjunctiva. Cyanosis indicates hypoxia.

Peripheral cyanosis: Inspect nail bed. Cyanosis can be due to vasoconstriction or hypoxia.

4.

The angle of attachment of the nail to the cuticle is greater than 180 degrees.

5.

- Do you have a history of skin cancer or other skin problems?
- Do you have a history of sun exposure?
- Do you have any medical problems, such as diabetes mellitus, cardiovascular disease, or endocrine problems?
- Do you have allergies?
- Are you on any medications? If so, what are they?

6.

Size, shape, location, drainage, texture, pedunculation, color, and tenderness

7.

Decreased skin elasticity, decreased sweat, atrophy and thinning of skin, and decreased pigmentation of skin and hair

8.

Seborrheic keratosis, keratotic horns, actinic keratosis, and age spots

9.

Asymmetry, border irregularity, color change or variegation, and diameter greater than 0.5 cm

10.

Temperature, hydration, elasticity, color, and odor

11.

Skin color changes may not be readily seen in dark skin, so assess the conjunctiva and oral mucosa for color changes.

12.

Are you on any medications?

Do you have any medical problems, such as thyroid disease?

Have you recently been seriously ill?

Do you have a family history of hair loss?

Do you use hair dyes or have permanents?

13.

For answers, see "Relationship of the Integumentary System to Other Systems," on page 142 of the text, and "Assessment of the Integumentary System's Relationship to Other Systems," on page 186 of the text.

14.

Age, dementia, incontinence and use of diapers, being bedridden, and restricted fluid intake

15.

Frail, lethargic, inattentive; temperature 101.2°F; wrinkled, loose skin with poor turgor; stage 1 pressure ulcers on heels and sacrum; and dusky blue nails

16.

Loose, wrinkled skin; poor skin turgor; gray hair; and increase in moles, cherry hemangiomas, and seborrheic keratosis

17.

a. Stage 1 pressure ulcers on heels and sacrum, immobility, inattentive/confused, possible dehydration, and incontinence

b. Restricted oral intake, temperature, poor skin turgor, and little urine output

c. Incontinent, uses diapers, and confusion

19.

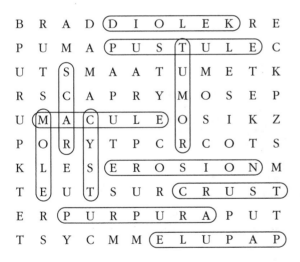

Chapter 9: Assessing the Head, Face, and Neck

1.

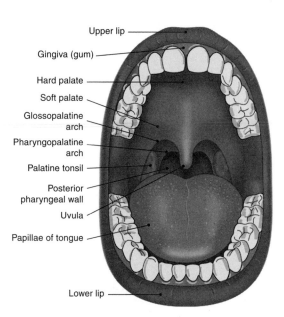

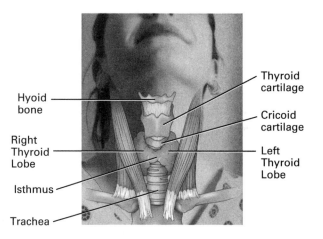

2.

1. b
2. d
3. g
4. f
5. j
6. h
7. c
8. l
9. i
10. a
11. e
12. k

3.

Red tonsils, exudates on tonsils, and enlarged tonsils

4.

20

5.

Color, condition, and bite

6.

Color, bleeding, and recession

7.

Tetracycline, because it causes discoloration of teeth

8.

Normal	Infection	Malignancy
≤ 1 cm	Enlarged	Enlarged
Round or oval	Round or oval	Irregular
Firm	Boggy	Hard
Movable	Movable	Fixed
Nontender	Tender	Nontender

9.

Trapezius and sterncleidomastoid

10.

Neutral, hyperextended, and as the person swallows

11.

Below the cricoid cartilage

12.

During pregnancy and puberty

13.

Palpating fontanels and measuring head circumference

14.

Nasolabial folds and palpebral fissures

15.

For answers, see "Relationship of the Head, Face, and Neck to Other Systems," on page 200 of the text, and "Assessment of the Head, Face, and Neck's Relationship to Other Systems," on page 237-238 of the text.

16.

Communication problem related to slurred speech, risk for stroke, TIA, family history of cerebrovascular accident, and risk for oral cancer related to history of smoking and chewing tobacco and positive family history of oral cancer

17.

HTN, TIA, carotid bruits, positive family history, being slightly overweight, and eating fried foods

18.

Speech difficulty, paralysis in right extremities, urinary incontinence, BP 186/108 mm Hg, decreased muscle strength on left side 4/5, movements clumsy, positive carotid bruits, and asymmetry of facial features

19.

Positive family history, positive smoking history and use of chewing tobacco, positive oral lesion and enlarged submandibular nodes, and weight loss

20.

Diet, HTN, stroke, oral cancer, and chewing tobacco

21.

a. Decreased motor function on left side of face, oral lesion, and unexplained weight loss
b. Risk for aspiration
c. Slurred speech.

23.

1. S (K) U L L

2. T H Y R (O) I D

3. U V U (L) A

4. S I N (U) S E S

5. C R (I) C O I D

6. T O N S I (L) S

7. T U R B I N (A) T E S

8. L Y M (P) H

9. T (E) E T H

10. G I N G I V (A)

11. N E C (K)

12. G O I T E R

K O (L) U I L A P E A K

A precancerous oral lesion is called LEUKOPLAKIA.

Chapter 10: Assessing the Eye and Ear

The Eye

1.

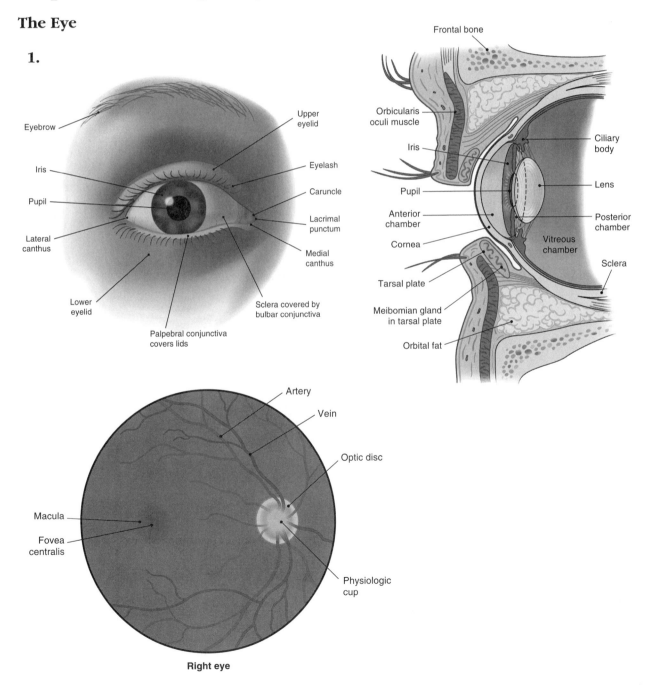

Right eye

2.

    1. f

    2. n

    3. d

    4. e

    5. m

    6. j

    7. k

    8. b

    9. c

    10. h

    11. a

    12. i

    13. g

    14. l

3.

OD 20/50: He can see at 20 feet what someone with normal far vision (20/20) could see at 50 feet with the right eye.

OS 20/40: He can see at 20 feet what someone with normal far vision could see at 40 feet with the left eye.

OU 20/40: He can see at 20 feet what someone with normal far vision could see at 40 feet with both eyes.

4.

No. Normal 20/20 vision is usually attained by the time the child reaches school age.

5.

Six cardinal fields of gaze test, cover/uncover test, and corneal light reflex test

6.

    1. c

    2. a

    3. b

    4. e

    5. d

    6. g

    7. f

7.

Darken the room, examine same eye to same eye, have the client look straight ahead, and always examine the macula last.

8.

    a. Used for undilated pupil

    b. Used for dilated pupil

    c. Used with fluorescein dye

    d. Filters red

    e. Locates lesions

    f. Used to determine shape of lesion

9.

For answers, see "Relationship of the Eyes and Ears to Other Systems," on page 251 of the text, and "Assessment of the Eyes' and Ears' Relationship to Other Systems," on page 283 of the text.

10.

What medications are you taking? She should not take mydriatic-producing medications because they dilate the pupil and increase intraocular pressure.

11.

Tonometry

12.

Blindness

13.

Her race—incidence of glaucoma is higher in African-Americans than in other races.

14.

    a. Complaint of severe eye pain

    b. Decreased peripheral vision and blurred vision

    c. Blurred vision, decreased peripheral vision, and colored halos

16.

    1. S(C)L E R A

    2. I R I S

    3. (M)E D I A L   C A N T H U S

    4. C O R N E A

    5. (L)A C R I M A L   G L A N D

    6. R E T I N A

    7. C O N J U N C T I V(A)

8. P (U) P I L

9. L E N S

10. F O V E (A)

C M L A U A

Always examine the MACULA last on funduscopic examination.

The Ear

1.

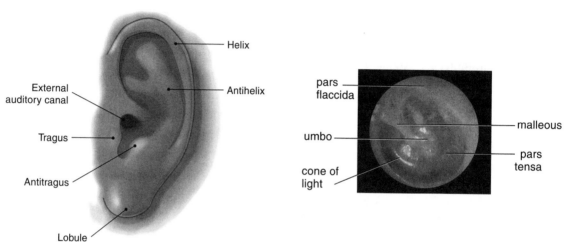

2.

1. c
2. d
3. h
4. g
5. a
6. b
7. e
8. f

3.

Do you have a history of frequent ear infections?

Are you taking any medications?

Have you ever had trauma to your ears?

Do you have a family history of hearing problems?

Are you exposed to noise pollution?

4.

With conductive hearing loss, the sound lateralizes to the bad ear. With sensorineural hearing loss, the sound lateralizes to the good ear.

5.

AC > BC; AC < BC

6.

Bloody drainage: Trauma

Purulent drainage: Infection

Clear/serous drainage: Allergies or CSF

7.

Tragus, mastoid, and helix (pull forward)

8.

Young child: Pull ear canal down.

Adult: Pull ear canal up and back.

9.

Color of tympanic membrane and external ear canal, position of landmarks, intactness of drum, and mobility of drum

10.

In a young child, the shape, size, and position of the ear canal and eustachian tubes—shorter, wider, and more horizontal—increase the risk for infection.

11.

For answers, see "Relationship of Eyes and Ears to Other Systems," on page 290 of text, and "Assessment of Eyes' and Ears' Relationship to Other Systems," on page 309 of text.

12.

Age, gender, history of recurrent ear infection, recent upper respiratory infection, and family history of otitis media

13.

Exposure to second-hand smoke and bottle-feeding

14.

Mobility of the drum

15.

a. Brian's complaint that "my ear hurts," tugging at ear, irritability, and tenderness of external ear

b. Recurrent ear infections

c. Fever and not eating well

d. Pain and not sleeping well

17.

1. O (T) I T I S   M (E) D I A

2. T (R) A G U S

3. M A S T O (I) D

4. I (N) C U S

5. M A L L (E) O L U S

6. S T (A) P E S

7. C (O) C H L E A

8. H E (L) I (X)

9. E X O (S)(T) O S I S

10. C H O L E S (T) E A T O M A

T E R I N E A O L X I S T T

Another name for swimmer's ear is EXTERNAL OTITIS.

Chapter 11: Assessing the Respiratory System

1.

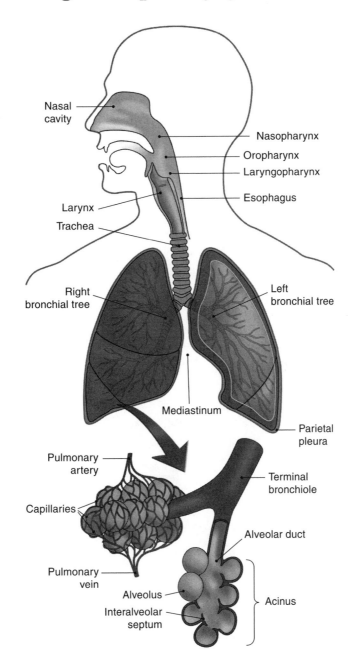

2.

1. c
2. e
3. f
4. b
5. a
6. d

3.

    1. j

    2. d

    3. i

    4. g

    5. c

    6. b

    7. a

    8. e

    9. h

    10. f

4.

Decreased breath sounds resulting from poor ventilatory effort, and shape of chest (e.g., musculoskeletal changes associated with aging)

5.

Peripheral cyanosis occurs in the periphery as a result of a localized problem or vasoconstriction. Central cyanosis results from hypoxia and is seen not only in the extremities, but also in the oral mucosa and conjunctiva.

6.

Change in mental status, confusion, or agitation

7.

Bronchial breath sounds over the affected lung with some crackles and rhonchi

8.

The right middle lobe is anatomically situated so that it can be assessed only from the anterior or lateral approach.

9.

Neurological system: Changes in mental status, such as confusion, irritability, and agitation

Integumentary system: Skin color changes, such as duskiness, pallor, or cyanosis; clammy skin

Cardiovascular system: Increased pulse rate and vasoconstriction

10.

For answers, see "Relationship of the Respiratory System to Other Systems," on page 316 of the text, and "Assessment of the Respiratory System's Relationship to Other Systems," on page 338 of the text.

11.

Upper respiratory infection

12.

Right congestive heart failure secondary to emphysema

13.

Signs/symptoms of hypoxia, including fatigue, shortness of breath, and central and peripheral cyanosis

14.

Emphysema can cause overinflation of lungs, which pushes diaphragm down to T12. Because lungs are overinflated, no change is seen when assessing diaphragmatic excursion.

15.

Barrel chest, costal angle greater than 90 degrees, pursed-lip breathing, shortness of breath, hyperresonance at bases, level of diaphragm at T12, and decreased breath sounds at bases

16.

a. Productive cough, foul-smelling yellow mucus, shortness of breath, respirations 28/min, and scattered rhonchi and wheezes

b. Shortness of breath, difficulty moving secretions, clubbing, pale gray mucous membranes, and reduced activity tolerance

c. Shortness of breath, decreased appetite, and being underweight

18.

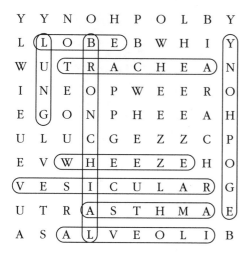

Chapter 12: Assessing the Cardiovascular System

1.

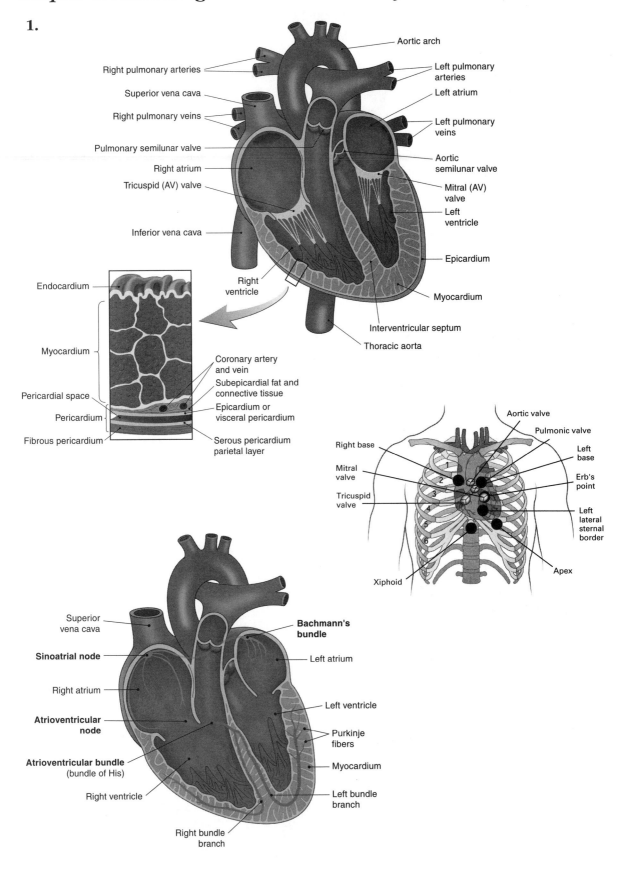

2.

　　1. f
　　2. g
　　3. e
　　4. o
　　5. m
　　6. b
　　7. h
　　8. c
　　9. a
　　10. i
　　11. l
　　12. n
　　13. j
　　14. k
　　15. d

3.

　　1. c
　　2. g
　　3. h
　　4. i
　　5. b
　　6. j
　　7. e
　　8. f
　　9. d
　　10. a

4.

S_1 is louder at the apex; S_2 is louder at the base.

5.

Split S_1 at tricuspid area; split S_2 at pulmonic area

6.

During inspiration, more blood returns to the right side of the heart than the left side. This means that the right side of the heart takes more time to pump, resulting in a split S_2 during inspiration.

7.

S_1 is loudest at apex; S_2 is loudest at base.
S_1 correlates with QRS of ECG.
S_1 precedes palpable carotid pulsation.

8.

S_4: Late diastolic sound heard when left atrium contracts against resistance.

9.

S_3: Early diastolic sound heard as blood rushes into a dilated, noncompliant left ventricle.

10.

Carotid pulsation is palpable; jugular pulsation is not.

Carotids have one upstroke; jugulars have an undulated wave.

Carotids are not affected by position; jugulars are.

Carotids are not affected by respirations; jugulars are.

11.

The sternal angle (angle of Louis) and the highest point of jugular venous pulsation

12.

a. Split S_1 from S_4: Split S_1 is a high-pitched systolic sound heard best at the left lower sternal border. An S_4 is a low-pitched diastolic sound heard best at the apex.

b. Split S_1 from ejection click: Split S_1 is a high-pitched systolic sound heard best at the left lower sternal border. An ejection click is a high-pitched mid-to-late systolic sound.

c. Split S_2 from S_3: Split S_2 is a high-pitched systolic sound heard best at base left during inspiration. S_3 is a low-pitched diastolic sound heard best at the apex.

d. Split S_2 from opening snap: Split S_2 is a high-pitched systolic sound heard best at base left during inspiration. An opening snap is a high-pitched systolic sound heard best at the apex.

13.

Pericardial friction rub—a high-pitched, scratchy sound heard best at the left lower sternal border.

14.

Increased flow through a normal valve, flow through a constricted valve, flow into a dilated chamber, shunting, and backflow through an incompetent valve

15.

Location heard, pitch, duration, quality, timing in cardiac cycle, and intensity

16.

Diastolic murmur or murmur greater than grade 3

17.

Have client hold breath; the bell

18.

For answers, see "Relationship of the Cardiovascular System of Other Systems," on page 371 of the text, and "Assessment of the Cardiovascular System's Relationship to Other Systems," on page 390-391 of the text.

19.

Cardiovascular and respiratory

20.

HTN and left ventricular hypertrophy

21.

Signs of right-sided heart failure

22.

S_4 could be associated with HTN or acute myocardial infarction, and S_3 could be associated with congestive heart failure.

23.

    a. Complains of chest discomfort; anxious, clutching chest; and elevated BP, pulse, and respirations

    b. Appears anxious; states, "Am I going to die?"; and has increase in vital signs

    c. Skin pale/ashen and diaphoretic; mucous membranes pale gray; capillary refill poor; skin cool, pale, shiny, and hairless on lower extremities; and +1 peripheral pulses

    d. Tachycardia with irregular rhythm; HTN; ECG shows anterior wall myocardial infarction, S_3, and S_4; skin ashen, cool, and diaphoretic; poor capillary refill; bibasilar crackles; neck vein distention and jugular venous pressure greater than 3 cm; and positive abdominal jugular reflux

24.

Decreased cardiac output and ineffective tissue perfusion. Improving cardiac output and tissue perfusion is essential to maintain life.

26.

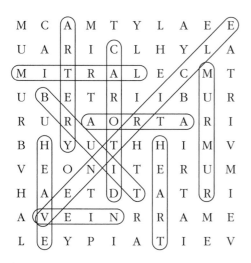

Chapter 13: Assessing the Peripheral-Vascular and Lymphatic Systems

1.

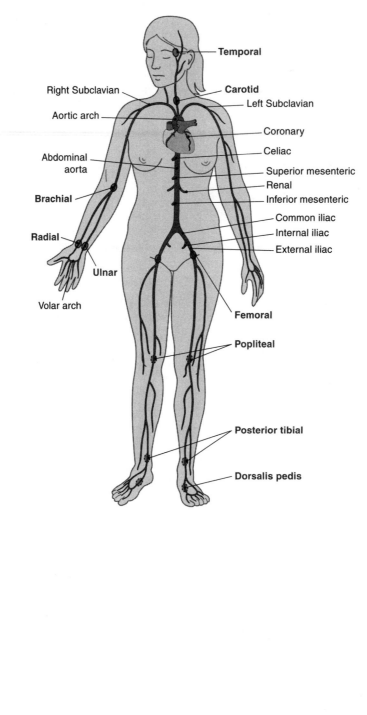

Temporal

Right Subclavian

Carotid

Left Subclavian

Aortic arch

Coronary

Celiac

Abdominal aorta

Superior mesenteric

Renal

Inferior mesenteric

Brachial

Common iliac

Internal iliac

Radial

External iliac

Ulnar

Volar arch

Femoral

Popliteal

Posterior tibial

Dorsalis pedis

2.

1. c
2. f
3. e
4. j
5. d
6. b
7. h
8. i
9. a
10. g

3.

As you inflate the cuff, palpate the brachial artery to the point at which the pulse is obliterated, then deflate the cuff. Reinflate the cuff 20 to 30 mm higher than the point at which the pulse was obliterated, and listen for BP.

4.

Supine, sitting, and standing

5.

BP: Systolic pressure drops 10 to 20 mm Hg.
Pulse: Pulse rate increases about 20 beats/min.
Level of consciousness: Client feels light-headed or faint.

6.

Rate, rhythm, contour, elasticity, amplitude, and equality

7.

Decreased elasticity

8.

Arterial insufficiency: Absent or decreased pulse; pallor or rubor; thin, hairless skin; and lesions on toes
Venous insufficiency: Edema; brownish discoloration; thick, leathery skin; and lesions on ankles

9.

Ankle-brachial index

10.

Size, shape, consistency, tenderness, and mobility

11.

Enlarged, round, boggy-to-firm, tender, mobile nodes

12.

Lymph nodes are biggest in childhood and get smaller with age.

13.

For answers, see "Relationship of the Peripheral-Vascular System to Other Systems," on page 413 of the text, and "Assessment of the Peripheral-Vascular System's Relationship to Other Systems," on page 426 of the text.

14.

History of HTN, diabetes mellitus, coronary artery disease, and smoking; family history of myocardial infarction and cerebrovascular accident

15.

Lesions on toes; absent pulses; thin, shiny skin on extremities, with patchy hair loss; thick nails; color changes in legs; and cool feet

16.

Ankle-brachial index

17.

Because blood flow must be adequate to the lower extremities to ensure healing.

18.

a. Intermittent claudication and cramping in legs when walking, relieved by rest
b. Intermittent claudication; cool feet; absent pedal pulses; thin, shiny skin and patchy hair loss on extremities; and color changes in legs
c. Ulcers on toes

20.

Diet, vascular disease, diabetes mellitus, HTN, and foot care

21.

Walking exercises for 15 to 30 minutes several times a day to improve collateral circulation

22.

Inspect feet daily, do not soak feet, keep feet clean and dry, wear shoes that fit properly, and have podiatrist cut toenails

23.

1. (B)R A C H I A L

2. K O R O (T)K O F F

3. B U E (R)G E R ' S   D I S E A S E

4. R A Y N A (U)D ' S   D I (S)E A S E

5. H O M A N ' S   S (I)G N

6. A L L E N   T E S T

7. P O P L I T E A L

8. F E M O R A L

9. V E I N

10. A R T E R Y

B T R U S I
Arteries are auscultated for BRUITS.

Chapter 14: Assessing the Breasts

1.

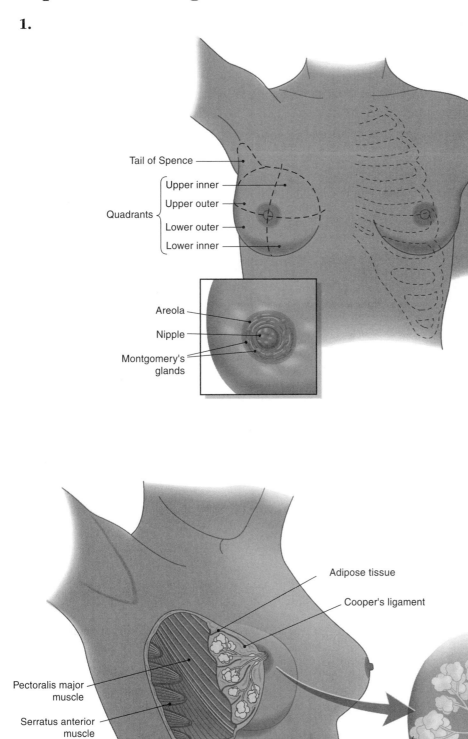

2.

    1. c

    2. d

    3. b

    4. e

    5. a

3.

Have you ever had breast cancer?

Do you have a family history of breast cancer?

Are you childless, or did you have your first child after age 30?

4.

On the fifth to seventh day of her menstrual cycle

5.

Sitting with hands at sides; sitting with hands over head; sitting with hands on hips; and standing, leaning forward

6.

Size, shape, consistency, mobility, and tenderness

7.

Increase in breast size and a mass that is hard, irregular in shape, and nonmobile and nontender

8.

    1. c

    2. d

    3. a

    4. b

9.

For answers, see "Relationship of the Breasts to Other Systems," on page 447 of the text, and "Assessment of the Breasts' Relationship to Other Systems," on page 464 of the text.

10.

Age, family history, race, early menarche, first full-term pregnancy after age 30

11.

Lymph nodes

12.

    a. Scheduled for lumpectomy

    b. Anxious, nervous, and tearful; states, "I'm so afraid it might be cancer."

    c. Scheduled for lumpectomy

14.

    1. P A G Ⓔ T ' S

    2. M Ⓐ S Ⓣ I T I S

    3. Ⓕ I B R Ⓞ A D E N O M A

    4. A R Ⓔ O Ⓛ A

    5. N Ⓘ P Ⓟ L E

    6. A Ⓒ I N I

    7. G Y Ⓝ E C O M A Ⓢ T I A

    E A T F O E L I P C N S

The most frequent site of breast cancer in women is the TAIL OF SPENCE.

Chapter 15: Assessing the Abdomen

1.

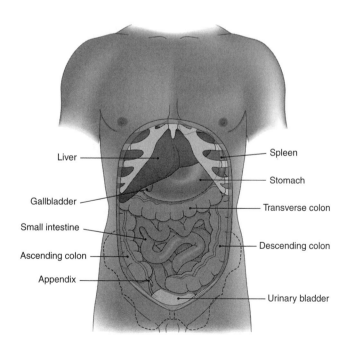

2.

    1. b

    2. d

    3. a

    4. c

    5. f

    6. e

    7. j

    8. g

    9. i

    10. h

3.

Liver: Right upper quadrant

Gallbladder: Right upper quadrant

Pancreas: Right upper quadrant and left upper quadrant

Stomach: Left upper quadrant

Spleen: Left upper quadrant

Cecum: Right lower quadrant

Appendix: Right lower quadrant

Sigmoid colon: Left lower quadrant

Transverse colon: Right upper quadrant, right lower quadrant, and left upper quadrant

Ascending colon: Right upper quadrant

Descending colon: Left upper quadrant and left lower quadrant

4.

    1. c

    2. a

    3. d

    4. e

    5. b

5.

Respirations, aortic pulsations, and peristalsis

6.

Palpation could alter bowel sounds.

7.

5 minutes

8.

Location: Right lower quadrant

Rationale: Active site; connects small and large intestine

9.

Effects of anesthesia, abdominal surgery, and decreased mobility

10.

Pain medication and immobility

11.

Diarrhea and early obstruction

12.

Scratch test

13.

Dullness

14.

6–12 cm

15.

No, the spleen needs to be about three times its normal size to be palpable.

16.

Midaxillary line

17.

For answers, see "Relationship of Abdomen to Other Systems," on page 493 of the text, and "Assessment of the Abdomen's Relationship to Other Systems," on page 495 of the text.

18.

A response to the pain. Shallow breathing minimizes abdominal movement.

19.

Time of last meal influences types of anesthesia or need for nasogastric tube to prevent aspiration if surgery is necessary.

20.

Do you have any allergies to drugs (e.g., penicillin), food, environmental factors, or latex?

21.

Temperature elevation: Inflammatory response, infection

Increased respirations: Response to pain

22.

Temperature elevation; increased, shallow respirations; guarding; decreased bowel sounds; tenderness in right lower quadrant; positive iliopsoas, Rovsing's, rebound, and obturator signs; cutaneous hypersensitivity signs; and body posture

23.

a. Statement of #10 pain in abdomen; guarding abdomen; shallow, increased respiratory rate; and high-normal range on pulse, temperature, and blood pressure

b. Statement about nausea and vomiting at home

c. Nausea, vomiting, and temperature elevation

24.

Apply ice bag to painful area, give nothing by mouth (NPO) in anticipation of upcoming surgery, give pain medications as ordered, and place client in semi-Fowler's position so that abdominal drainage can collect in lower quadrants.

25.

Muscle rigidity over entire abdomen; elevated BP, pulse, respiratory rate, and temperature; states that abdominal pain is worse with movement and coughing and better when flexing right hip and knee; abdomen is rigid or boardlike; bowel sounds are diminished.

27.

1. L I V E Ⓡ

2. Ⓟ E R I S T A L S I S

3. Ⓢ Ⓣ R I A E

4. Ⓜ E L E N A

5. F L A T Ⓤ S

6. Ⓒ H Y M E

7. Ⓑ O R B O R Ⓨ G M I

8. A S C I T E S

9. D I A R R H Ⓔ A

10. M A S T I C A T I Ⓞ Ⓝ

11. S P L E E Ⓝ

12. C Ⓘ R R H O S I S

R P S T M U C B Y E O N N I

The area of tenderness in acute appendicitis is MCBURNEY'S POINT.

Chapter 16: Assessing the Female Genitourinary System

1.

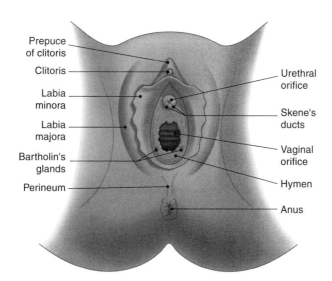

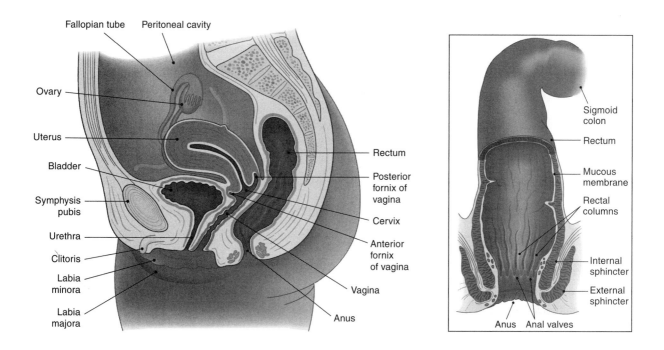

2.

   1. g

   2. f

   3. h

   4. i

   5. j

   6. d

   7. k

   8. l

   9. c

  10. e

  11. b

  12. a

3.

Decreased, irregular, or absent menses; hot flashes; and decreased vaginal secretions

4.

At age 18, or when she becomes sexually active

5.

A test for cervical cancer

6.

At what age did your menstrual periods start?

Can you describe your cycle? How often do you menstruate? How many days per month? How much do you bleed?

Do you use pads or tampons?

Are you sexually active?

If yes, do you practice safe sex? Do you use birth control?

7.

16 years

8.

To assess the reproductive organs (uterus, ovaries, cervix, and vagina), to detect any lesions, and to obtain specimens

9.

Parous: Os appears as a slit.

Nulliparous: Os appears round and closed.

10.

    1. b

    2. f

    3. e

    4. a

    5. h

    6. j

    7. k

    8. l

    9. m

   10. g

   11. c

   12. d

   13. i

11.

For answers, see "Relationship of Female Genitourinary System to Other Systems" on page 525 of the text and "Assessment of the Female Genitourinary System," on page 540 of the text.

12.

Vague abdominal complaints, change in bowel habits, loss of appetite, and weight loss but increase in abdominal girth

13.

Menarche age 11, nulliparous, age and race, fatty diet, and family history of ovarian cancer

14.

The respiratory system because ascites may push up the diaphragm and impinge respirations

15.

    a. Progressive vague abdominal complaints

    b. Change in bowel pattern; reports constipation

    c. Affect anxious; states she is "scared about what the doctor will find"

16.

    a. Surgical incision is a break in skin, the first line of defense

    b. Ascites may push diaphragm up and impinge respirations. Anesthesia may lead to hypoventilation. Pain may lead to hypoventilation.

18.

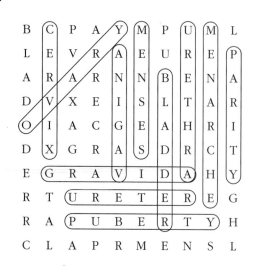

```
B  C  P  A  Y  M  P  U  M  L
L  E  V  R  A  E  U  R  E  P
A  R  A  R  N  B  R  E  N  A
D  V  X  E  I  L  E  T  A  R
O  I  A  C  G  A  T  H  R  I
D  X  G  R  A  S  D  R  C  T
E  G  R  A  V  I  D  A  H  Y
R  T  U  R  E  T  E  R  E  G
R  A  P  U  B  E  R  T  Y  H
C  L  A  P  R  M  E  N  S  L
```

Chapter 17: Assessing the Male Genitourinary System

1.

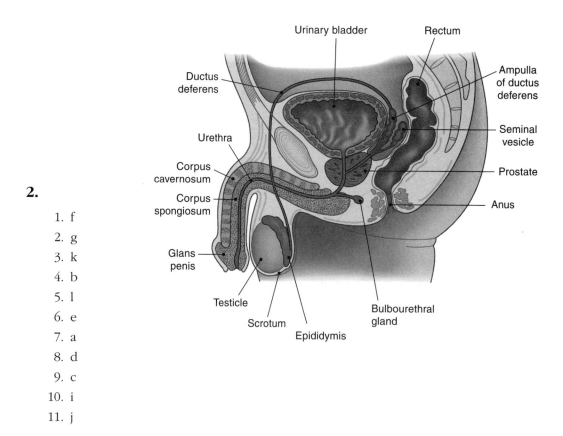

- Urinary bladder
- Rectum
- Ductus deferens
- Ampulla of ductus deferens
- Urethra
- Seminal vesicle
- Corpus cavernosum
- Prostate
- Corpus spongiosum
- Anus
- Glans penis
- Testicle
- Scrotum
- Epididymis
- Bulbourethral gland

2.

1. f
2. g
3. k
4. b
5. l
6. e
7. a
8. d
9. c
10. i
11. j

3.

    1. c

    2. j

    3. a

    4. l

    5. d

    6. h

    7. e

    8. i

    9. g

   10. b

   11. f

   12. k

4.

Risk factors are cryptorchidism and exposure to diethylstilbestrol (DES).

TSE should be done monthly.

Testicles should be egg-shaped and feel rubbery, firm, mobile, and nontender.

5.

Age 40

Prostatic-specific antigen test and digital rectal examination

6.

Alcohol and drug abuse, smoking, medications, and medical problems such as diabetes and cardiovascular disease

7.

Indirect and direct inguinal hernias and femoral hernias

8.

For answers, see "Relationship of the Male Genitourinary System to Other Systems," on page 562 of the text, and "Assessment of the Male Genitourinary System's Relationship to Other Systems," on page 575 of the text.

9.

Maintain open line of communication and remain nonjudgmental.

Determine through questioning what client knows about HIV and other STDs.

Perform physical examination.

Obtain STD screening tests and HIV test, explaining limitations of tests.

Discuss possible outcomes and potential interventions.

Provide education about STD prevention.

10.

Multiple sex partners, frequent sex with inconsistent use of condoms, excessive alcohol use, marijuana use, and history of STDs

11.

Condyloma (human papillomavirus)

12.

Use of condoms, types of STDs, and drug and alcohol use

13.

   a. Unprotected sexual activity, drug and alcohol use, and multiple sex partners
   b. Unprotected sexual activity, multiple partners, and risky behavior with drugs and alcohol
   c. Unprotected sexual activity and multiple partners

15.

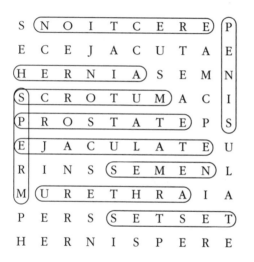

Chapter 18: Assessing the Musculoskeletal System

1.

   1. e
   2. c
   3. d
   4. g
   5. f
   6. a
   7. b

2.

    a. Hinge

    b. Ball and socket

    c. Condyloid

    d. Gliding/plane

    e. Hinge

    f. Ball and socket

    g. Saddle

3.

    1. d

    2. h

    3. b

    4. l

    5. m

    6. c

    7. j

    8. e

    9. f

    10. k

    11. a

    12. i

    13. g

4.

Standing and bending over, or "dive" position

5.

Cervical, thoracic, lumbar, and sacral

6.

Kyphosis: Accentuated thoracic curve

Scoliosis: Lateral deviation of spine

Lordosis: Accentuated lumbar curve

7.

- Arm length: Measure from acromium process to tip of middle finger
- Leg length: Measure from anterior superior iliac crest to medial malleolus

8.

Back pain, gait problem, and an apparent scoliosis

9.

If right arm is dominant side, circumference may be greater because of activity, such as sports.

10.

Stride length, base of support, conformity of phases, arm swing, toe position, and cadence

11.

Short stride length, wide base of support, and problems with phases (e.g., swing phase cadence may not be rhythmic)

12.

Wide base of support and shortened stride length

13.

Kyphosis

14.

ROM, deformity, redness, swelling, crepitus, pain, and stability

15.

5 = normal; 4 = movement against some resistance; 3 = movement against gravity with no resistance.

16.

Observe gait; have client hop on one foot, tandem walk (heel to toe), heel and toe walk, and do deep knee bends; and perform Romberg's test.

17.

- Upper: Rapid alternating movements and finger-thumb opposition
- Lower: Toe tapping and heel down shin

18.

Point-to-point localization and finger to nose

19.

For answers, see "Relationship of the Musculoskeletal System to Other Systems," on page 595 of the text, and "Assessment of the Relationship of the Musculoskeletal System to Other Systems," on page 608 of the text.

20.

Age, weight, and occupation

21.

Her occupation

22.

a. Pain in lower back when sitting or lying for extended periods. "Feels like a dull knife in my lower back, I usually get up and walk around to relieve it. It's my bones; they are getting old." Rates pain as 7 on 1-to-10 scale. Diagnosed with DJD 2 years ago, which has been getting progressively worse.
b. Cannot sit or stand for prolonged periods without developing pain

24.

1. B O N Ⓔ

2. Ⓣ E N D O N

3. L Ⓘ G A M E Ⓝ T

4. Ⓛ U M B A R

5. S Ⓟ I N E

6. B A L A Ⓝ C E

7. S A C R A Ⓛ

8. T Ⓗ O R A C I C

9. G Ⓐ I T

10. M U S C L Ⓔ

E T I N L P N L H A E
Two tests for carpal tunnel syndrome are the TINEL and PHALEN tests.

Chapter 19: Assessing the Sensory-Neurological System

1.

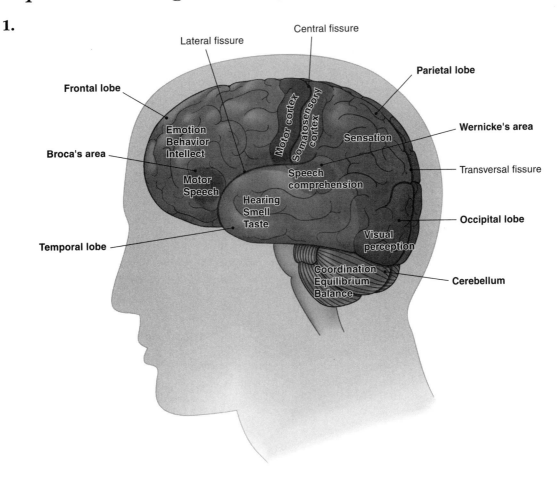

2.

1. b
2. l
3. j
4. c
5. a
6. h
7. f
8. e
9. g
10. k
11. i
12. d

3.

Person, place, and time

4.

Sternal rub, nail pressure, and Achilles pinch

5.

Nipple twist and eyeball pressure

6.

Immediate, recent, and remote memory

7.

Immediate and recent

8.

Psychiatric problem

9.

1. c
2. a
3. b
4. e
5. d
6. j
7. f
8. g
9. h
10. l
11. i
12. k

10.

1. b
2. e
3. d
4. a
5. c

11.

Have the client clench his or her teeth or interlock the hands and push.

12.

0 = absent; +1 = diminished; +2 = normal; +3 = hyperactive; +4 = hyperactive with clonus.

13.

Normal: Toe curling
Abnormal: Fanning of toes and dorsiflexion of great toe

14.

Close your eyes.

15.

Temperature, because pain and temperature run along the same tract

16.

Yes for deep sensation, no for superficial sensation

17.

Have the client close his or her eyes, then place a vibrating tuning fork on a bony prominence on a finger and a toe.

18.

Have the client close his or her eyes, then move your finger up and down and ask the client to identify the direction of movement.

19.

1. c
2. e
3. d
4. b
5. a

20.

For answers, see "Relationship of the Sensory-Neurological System to Other Systems," on page 651 of the text, and "Assessment of the Sensory-Neurological System's Relationship to Other Systems," on page 688 of the text.

21.

Increased intracranial pressure

22.

A change in level of consciousness

23.

Worsening headache, vomiting, sleepy, lethargic, change in Glasgow Coma Scale to 14, change in pupillary reaction (sluggish), change in vital signs, widening pulse pressure, decrease in heart rate, and decrease in motor strength

24.

a. Headache and vomiting, change in level of consciousness, change in pupils, and change in vital signs
b. Involved in car accident and sustained concussion, complaints of worsening headache, and guarding head and neck

26.

1. B R Ⓐ I N

2. ⒸO R T E X

3. T H A Ⓛ A M U S

4. ⓈY N A P S E

5. A F F Ⓔ R E N T

6. N E U R O N Ⓢ

7. C E R E B E Ⓛ L U M

8. M E D U L L Ⓐ

9. ⓌE R N I C K E

10. B R Ⓞ C A ' S Ⓐ R E A

11. ⒼR A Y ⓂA T T E R

12. ⒸE R E B R U M

13. M E N I N Ⓖ E S

14. ⓄC C I P I T A L L O B E

A C L S E S L A W O A G M C G O

The universal tool used to assess level of consciousness is the GLASGOW COMA SCALE.

Chapter 20: Putting It All Together

1.

Cardiovascular examination and TSE

2.

HTN, cardiovascular disease, diet (especially cholesterol), and occupational safety

3.

Positive: Sought health screening; has supports

Negative: Smoking, alcohol use, high-cholesterol diet, family history of cardiovascular disease, occupational risks, doesn't practice preventive screenings

4.

a. Lack of ability to perform TSE

b. Construction worker

Chapter 21: Assessing the Mother-to-Be

1.

1. e
2. g
3. l
4. k
5. m
6. h
7. b
8. n
9. a
10. d
11. f
12. c
13. i
14. o
15. j

2.

   a. Positive

   b. Presumptive

   c. Probable

   d. Presumptive

   e. Probable

   f. Probable

   g. Presumptive

   h. Presumptive

   i. Probable

   j. Probable

   k. Positive

   l. Probable

   m. Presumptive

   n. Presumptive

   o. Presumptive

3.

Diabetes, HTN, mitral valve prolapse, hepatitis B, cancer, rubella, and STDs

4.

Weight, fundal height, fetal heart tones, and fetal position

5.

7/8/03

6.

Breasts, fundus, bleeding, vascular assessment for thrombus, urination, episiotomy or incision, and gastrointestinal problems such as hemorrhoids and bowel movements

7.

For answers, see "Normal Changes Associated with Pregnancy," on pages 714-719 of the text.

9.

Soft uterus, heavy bleeding, pale color, and vital signs

10.

Low BP, increased pulse, pale color, poor capillary refill, skin cool and clammy, soft uterus, and heavy bleeding with clots

11.

Shallow respirations, decreased sensation in lower extremities, weakness, and numbness of lower extremities

12.

Skin turgor, hydration, mucous membranes, and urinary output

13.

The abdomen

14.

Supports, prenatal classes, instructions on infant care and breast-feeding, and follow-up care for mother and infant

15.

    a. Heavy bleeding, low BP, increased pulse, pale color, and cool and clammy skin
    b. Type of anesthesia, hypoventilating, and tender abdominal incision
    c. Cesarean section and surgical incision
    d. Surgery and abdominal incision

Chapter 22: Assessing the Newborn

1.

    1. k
    2. c
    3. a
    4. f
    5. d
    6. e
    7. l
    8. b
    9. j
    10. h
    11. i
    12. g

2.

Heart rate, respirations, muscle tone, color, and reflex irritability (cry)

3.

Prenatal history; pregnancy, labor, and delivery; anesthesia; type of delivery; medication use during pregnancy (including alcohol, illegal drugs, and OTC drugs); medical problems during pregnancy; and prenatal care

4.

Head, chest, abdomen, length, and weight

5.

1. d
2. g
3. l
4. b
5. k
6. e
7. f
8. p
9. j
10. m
11. h
12. i
13. c
14. o
15. n
16. a

6.

For answers, see "Performing a Head-to-Toe Physical Assessment," on pags 754-765 of the text.

8.

Age—commonly occurs between 1 and 10 weeks of age

Gender—more common in boys

Race—more common in whites than blacks or Asians

Being full-term—more common in full-term infants than premature infants

Family history of pyloric stenosis

Birth order—more common in firstborns

9.

How many bowel movements does he have a day? What are their color and consistency?

How many diaper changes does he need a day for urination?

How many times a day does he vomit, and how much?

How many feedings is he able to keep down a day?

10.

Vomiting within 1 hour after feeding, projectile vomiting, vomitus described as stale milk, distended upper abdomen, reverse peristaltic waves, and palpable olive-shaped mass in epigastric region

11.

Vomiting; weight loss; increase in temperature, pulse, and respirations; sunken fontanels; dry, warm skin and mucous membranes; and lethargic, weak, and inactive

12.

Trust versus mistrust

13.

Allow mother to stay with child

14.

a. Vomiting; increase in vital signs; sunken fontanels; dry, warm skin and mucous membranes; and weight loss
b. Weight loss and vomiting

15.

Secondary to vomiting

Chapter 23: Assessing the Toddler and Preschooler

1.

Successful: Gains control over bodily functions, can separate from parents, is able to differentiate self from others, can tolerate delayed gratification
Unsuccessful: Feels shame and doubt, has temper tantrums, persistently says "no"

2.

Successful: Develops conscience, sees actions as good or bad, motivated by reward or punishment
Unsuccessful: Is unable to see actions as good or bad

3.

Toilet training, temper tantrums, and accidents

4.

Repeated ED visits, physical findings that are inconsistent with stated cause of injury, inappropriate response by child or parent, inconsistent accounts of injury, other signs of abuse, and evidence of old abuse

5.

Allow parent to be with child, use toys or games to demonstrate parts of examination, and do otoscope/ophthalmoscope examination last

6.

Need to measure head circumference, plot height and weight on growth charts, assess fontanel, and pull ear lobe down when performing the otoscopic examination

7.

For answers, see "Performing a Head-to-Toe Physical Assessment," on pages 789-793 of the text.

9.

Low weight and small size for age; 24-hour dietary recall

10.

Diet mainly consists of bottles of milk.

11.

History of recurrent ear infections, recent upper respiratory infection, his age, bottles at bedtime, and exposure to secondhand smoke

12.

Lead paint poisoning; motor vehicle injuries due to improper car seat

13.

History of recurrent ear infections, recent upper respiratory infection, fever, tugging at ear, irritable, not sleeping well, decreased appetite, red tympanic membrane, and lymphadenopathy

14.

Not active, increased heart rate and respirations, pale conjunctiva, spoon-shaped nails, 24-hour dietary recall shows nutritional deficits, and low hematocrit and hemoglobin

15.

Fever, dehydration, and anemia

16.

Max's diet, bottles at bedtime, exposure to secondhand smoke, possible lead paint exposure, car safety

17.

Autonomy versus shame and doubt

18.

Bowel and bladder control

19.

24-hour dietary recall and nutritional deficits

20.

   a. Temperature elevation: 101.2°F (rectal)

   b. Age, dietary deficits, and anemia

   c. Old house with probable exposure to lead paint, and improper car safety

Chapter 24: Assessing the School-Age Child and Adolescent

1.

Successful: Develops independence, learns to work and cooperate with others, builds relationships outside home with peers and teachers, develops a conscience

Unsuccessful: Is dependent; fails in school; has difficulty developing relationships; engages in unhealthy, risky behaviors

2.

Successful: Develops a sense of self and self-competency and a set of personal values, plans for future career.

Unsuccessful: Develops poor self-image, is insecure, engages in unhealthy, risky behaviors

3.

Sports-related injuries, motor vehicle accidents, substance abuse, eating disorders, and sexual activity

4.

Substance abuse (drugs, alcohol, and smoking); injuries (use of safety equipment when engaging in sports); automobile/driving safety; nutrition (obesity/eating disorders); and sexuality, including STDs and pregnancy

5.

Height and weight are compared on growth charts, and secondary sexual characteristic development is assessed.

6.

For answers, see "Performing a Head-to-Toe Physical Assessment," on pages 803-806 of the text.

8.

Weakness and fatigue, color pale, mucous membranes pale, increase in pulse, low BP and respirations, positive systolic murmur II/VI, bleeding gums, and bruises

9.

Temperature elevation, lymph node enlargement, and fatigue

10.

a. Risk for infection related to compromised immune system

b. Risk for injury related to bone marrow effects

c. Risk for volume fluid deficit related to bleeding

11.

a. Weight loss, loss of appetite, and acute lymphocytic leukemia

b. Complaints of fatigue

13.

Industry versus inferiority

14.

Needs to have sense of accomplishments in school and develop relationships outside of home

15.

The amount she exercises would lead you to think she has a low lean:fat ratio that contributes to amenorrhea.

16.

Exercise regimen, and irregular cycles are common for 1 to 2 years after menarche

17.

Secondary

18.

History of anemia, weight loss

19.

Identity versus role diffusion

20.

Develop relationships, career choices

21.

   a. Height in 5% and weight in less than 5%
   b. Unaware that exercise pattern has effect on menstrual cycle

Chapter 25: Assessing the Older Adult

1.

Multiple problems with multiple treatments, differing disease presentation in the elderly, and exaggeration of symptoms by client if he or she is a "health pessimist"

2.

Allow more time; ask about hearing problems; speak slowly, clearly, and with a low pitch; redirect, but realize the older client's need to reminisce

3.

Successful: Satisfaction with life, sense of contributing to society
Unsuccessful: Depression, alcohol abuse, suicidal

4.

Keep environment warm and well lit, but use nonglaring light; keep background noise down; use higher than standard seating for client; and minimize position changes

5.

For answers, see "Performing a Head-to-Toe Physical Assessment," on pages 843-854 of the text.

6.

 1. b
 2. c
 3. d
 4. a

8.

Integrity versus despair

9.

The pain and decreased ability to be active could lead to depression.

10.

Rheumatoid arthritis is systemic, with associated symptoms of fatigue and fever.

11.

Age, occupation, and weight

12.

Pain with movement, limited ROM, gait problems, crepitus, decreased strength, and swelling of knees

13.

 a. Pain increases with activity
 b. Knee pain, decreased ROM, needs cane to walk, and decreased strength
 c. Reports awakening at night with knee pain